Foundations of Energy Healing

The Essential Guide for Opening into the Quantum Field

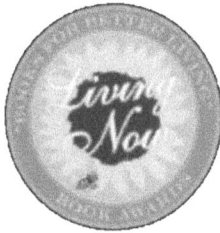

FOUNDATIONS OF ENERGY HEALING

THE ESSENTIAL GUIDE FOR OPENING INTO THE QUANTUM FIELD

Randi Botnick

Radiant Heart Press
Milwaukee, Wisconsin

Published by
Radiant Heart Press
An imprint of HenschelHAUS Publishing, Inc.
www.henschelHAUSbooks.com

ISBN: 978-1-59598-931-4
LCCN: 2015951946

Originally published as *4th Dimensional Healing: A Guidebook for a New Paradigm of Healing.* in 2015 under ISBN 978-1-59598-432-6

Cover design by Dan Fleming
Author photo by Kat Forder Photography

Printed in the United States of America

Illustration credits:
Flower of Life © Forbfruit | Dreamstime.com
Globe & Flower of Life © Peter Hermes Furian & Forbfruit| Dreamstime.com
Meridians – Front © Steve Allen | Dreamstime.com
Meridians – Back © Steve Allen | Dreamstime.com
Etheric Energy Body © Robin Shotola (used on cover and in the book)
Chakra Icons © Peter Hermes Furian | Dreamstime.com
Hands © Robin Shotola
Lymph System (body outline) © AlexanderZam | Dreamstime.com & Robin Shotola
Run Lymph System (body outline) © AlexanderZam | Dreamstime.com

To the searchers, seekers,
healers, and mystics.
(You know who you are.)

Dare to be authentic!

Table of Contents

Acknowledgements

Thank you, thank you, thank you to all of my past and present clients for your trust, support and loyalty over the years. I love you all!

My gratitude goes out to Leslie Jessica Palmer and Christel Libiot, who gave me wonderful feedback, editing and, most of all, the support only girlfriends can give. I also want to thank Kira Henschel from the bottom of my heart for making this publication possible with her expertise and patience.

Finally, I want to thank the Federation of Councils for all of their collaboration, inspiration, and encouragement throughout this process. The Federation came to me in channelings and meditations more than a year before this book, and I am forever grateful to them for their guidance and unconditional Love from start to finish.

Preface

*What if that which we perceive with our five senses
was only a small piece of all there is to experience?*

I started practicing healing work in 1997 when I became a
Reiki practitioner. I put up a flyer on the local Whole Foods'
bulletin board, and, lo and behold!, people called me. I
studied and practiced and studied and practiced for years, always
curious, and wanting to understand more. I asked, *What is energy
exactly? How does this work? What else can I do with this?*

And always, *"Who is it who is helping me?"*

Like so many others before me, I have been living my life for
the past twenty years in two seemingly disparate worlds, firmly
planted in the perceived reality of the third-dimensional world,
with occasional glimpses into the existence of the higher-
dimensional reality, receiving assistance from many Lightbeings—
angels, ascended masters, and alien beings. It is just a part of my
personality that, when I had metaphysical and spiritual experiences, I never doubted them. However, it took me many years to
incorporate them fully into my experience because I had few
teachers and colleagues who could verify and validate my
experiences.

My goal with this book is to help energy healers integrate the
experiences of the fourth—and fifth—dimensions into their
healing practices, and ultimately, into daily life. My intention is not
to prove to you that my perceptions are real, but to support you
and help your perceptions expand into an ever greater awareness
of what *is*. This is the book I would have liked to have had access
to when my extrasensory gifts were beginning to emerge: a

practical guide that illustrates the mystical and metaphysical possibilities of healing.

> *In 2006, I was working on a client in my office. During the session, I saw a being standing at the far end of the table, working on my client's lower body. I saw his "hands," which looked bizarrely like bug claws. He wore a cloak, and his face was covered. I could barely make it out. I felt his energy, which was soft and loving, even though I had the impression that his physical appearance was far from soft. At the end of the session, I thanked him for his presence and he bowed to me.*

> *After the session, I moved on, forgetting about him, until the next time he came in, which he began to do often. I kept asking to see his face, but he declined, psychically letting me know that most humans are afraid of it. We continued on that way for many weeks, until finally, after asking many times, he dropped the hood and showed me his face—a long, dog-like nose covered in leathery skin.*

> *I understood immediately that he was an alien being, a healer, coming to help. He was my assistant, an extra set of hands that added greater power and higher knowledge to the session. I felt nothing but love from, and for, him. I came to expect his presence during my healings, but never spoke about him to anyone in between sessions.*

I had read many books on energy healing, most of which were written in the late nineties and were about Therapeutic Touch and Reiki. I had also read many spiritual books about angels and spirit guides. What I did not have when I was first learning was a book that incorporated all of that for me, thereby validating my own experiences. I felt as if I was blazing my own trail, which was difficult for me personally and professionally. Had I had more access to what had been experienced before me, I believe I would have been able to progress more smoothly in my abilities and my process.

Preface

Many people to whom I have taught Reiki ask me questions about whether or not they can trust their experiences when they receive unexpected spiritual guidance. And as there seems to be no foundational framework or common language in our culture for metaphysical experiences, having some kind of confirmation from other people is very helpful.

This kind of spiritual guidance, in the form of energy, information and Light, is more accessible to us now than ever before. We live in a time when we are transitioning out of the shells of the physical third-dimensional world and into a new awareness of the multi-dimensional world. As the entire world makes this transition, all beings are "waking up" a little bit more. This awakening causes old, fear-based vibrations that no longer serve us to rise to the surface, like oil in water. The discomfort this is creating is leading more and more people to find ways to heal themselves. Likewise, Lightworkers (those of us who volunteered, before birth, to help the planet and its population heal from the effects of fear) are feeling the call to go to work in this arena.

Our spirit guides and the Lightbeings are committed to helping us shed the illusions that block us from that aim. All of us on the planet now are destined to begin this ascension process in this lifetime. We are all worthy of this.

The following list was given to us by Kryon, a loving, angelic energy, via Lee Carroll in a channeled message in 2014. For more than 26 years, the loving information from their partnership has sustained many and explained much about our changing time.

> *"Human nature is about to shift and it will be the first time in any of your history where this has happened...You are entering into a new energy that has never been here before, and these attributes of what is happening will eventually change Human nature itself. It's going to change everything about you, and civilization on the planet... This will be an evolution taking you to a new place that has not existed before—*

Foundations of Energy Healing

*a wisdom the earth has never seen, and a slow building
of a new kind of harmonious peace on the planet."*

Our five senses deceive us to create an illusion of separation—a
fact that I will refer to in this book over and over again. This is
merely the third-dimensional game that we have all been playing,
one of imagining ourselves to be separate from the Source of All
That Is, for the sole (soul?) purpose of experiencing the joy of
re-membering. Is this too hard to believe?

Here is an example of how our senses deceive us. Our
elementary senses tell us that the world is flat—it looks and feels
flat. We operated under that false perception for millennia. It took
some free thinkers (beginning in the 15th century) to convince us
otherwise, and, of course, scientific advancements have shown us
that our Earth is round.

It is becoming an imperative to learn to trust and recognize
the language of our sixth sense. Whether you call it intuition,
psychic perceptions, or gut feelings—the sixth sense is as real as
the other five, and everyone can attune to it. To do so, one must
leave the conscious, analytical mind and enter into a more subtle
sense of the body. Yet the paradox is that we perceive the subtle
world primarily through feeling, seeing, and hearing, as well as
through pure knowing. As these perceptions open and grow,
many begin to wonder if they are crazy. I believe that it may be
crazier to live only in the world of the third-dimensional physical
reality, which blocks out potentially ninety percent of our true
nonmaterial existence.

It is nearly impossible to translate into words the experiences
of the subtle world; therefore, we barely have the language to
describe this poorly understood science of psychic phenomena. In
this book, I verbalize that which is without form. I express what
may seem improbable: that we truly have access to all the help
and healing we are ready for at any given time.

No two people will have the same perceptions or information
coming in. Everyone gets it in a way that makes sense to her. The
pictures I see are my own interpretations of the energy and

information that comes to me, and your perception is specific to you.

All of this makes the information shared here not yet able to be proven scientifically; yet it is an accurate representation of my experience. This book is not meant to tell you what to do. If you have questions, this book may have the answers. But if you were already doing things that work well for you, that is perfect. My intention here is not to ask you to become me and do what I do, but to allow you to open up to the greatest possibilities of who you truly and authentically are, and help you realize that you can heal and help others heal, too!

In this book, I will cover:

- What it means to connect to the higher dimensions to access our spiritual and extra-sensory healing gifts;

- An explanation of healing from the perspective of being multidimensional beings in a multidimensional world;

- How to facilitate sessions with clients;

- What to expect as the healer—the conduit of the subtle energies;

- What to expect from the spiritual healing team—the beings who assist us with this process;

- How to clear trauma issues; and

- Energy clearing processes.

As a purchaser of this book, you automatically have access to recordings of meditations, visualizations and processes in the Self-Help Tools and Emotional Release Processes. Each is available in a male and a female voice to match your preference. You can listen to or download the recordings at www.4dhealingguide.com.

The words *energy*, *Light*, *information* and *intelligence* are used interchangeably, as all of these words describe the same phenomena. I understand that sometimes the connotation of each of these words means something different to different people, but my intention is to assert that they are one in the same.

I use the words *Source, Source Creator* and *God* interchangeably as well.

1. The Great Awakening

What if we were walking around thinking
we are wide awake, but we are actually sleepwalking?

Agreat shift is taking place on our planet. The earth's
energy is rising in vibration. We are all feeling it on some
level, from the subtlest sense of discomfort with how life
has been up until now, to the most surprising changes such as the
emergence of new psychic and paranormal gifts.

Our world is waking up to multiple dimensions of reality. All
along, we have been living in the third dimensional reality, a
purposeful state of perceived separation from everything around
us, including Source. This reality creates experiences of polarities:
right and wrong, better and worse, light and dark. And as we, as
spiritual beings, have perceived ourselves as separate, forgetting
ourselves to be the divine expressions of Source Creator, we have
been in a constant struggle to understand our powers and
freedoms.

In third-dimensional reality, the notion of God (or Source) is
based on a judgmental world. Life is about reward and punishment, and everyone and everything around us is a reflection of
that. In the third dimension, we believe only what we see — and
what we see looks separate and distinct.

Over time, our discernment has matured to include the ideas
that there is a connection between the Self and everything outside
of the self and that life is a co-creative experience. Life is about
cause and effect, and each one of us is responsible for his own
experiences. Within that, each experience is part of a whole, with
all facets originating from the vibration of Love, so on an

energetic level, no experience is better or worse than any other—although physically, some experiences can seem bad or painful.

We have awakened to the idea that there is more to this world than meets the eye (and ear). For some of us, the concepts of God and other spiritual beings have expanded as well. God is no longer presumed to be about reward and punishment. Instead, God is an essence, a life-force energy, found in and of everything. Because of this awareness, the heart chakra begins to expand and people feel more unconditionally loved and protected.

Each dimension we expand into is a different vibrational state that perpetuates certain perceptions and attitudes. In a higher dimensional awareness, people wake up to spiritual experiences that include insights and information from other beings. Intuition develops more fully, stimulating expansions of the five senses to perceive what is not on the physical plane, increasing empathy, precognition, dreams and healing abilities. Connections are made with angelic beings, elementals and alien races.

As we continue our expansion into even higher dimensions of awareness—an even higher vibration—we will open the door to unconditional love and acceptance. People will surrender completely to the Source Creator, with the understanding that self and God are not separate, but part of the same whole. Equality, unity, community and mastery are the perceptions of these higher dimensions.

This movement from one perspective to another, higher vibrational perspective, can be seen beginning to emerge in the 1960s, as many people began to question norms with the resulting social, civic and political dissonance. The transition gained momentum in the 1970s with the self-help movement and has continued into the present. During the 1970s, people felt allowed to begin "searching for themselves" in ways they were never allowed to do before. During that decade we witnessed a rise in personal transformation practices such as self-awareness, self improvement, yoga, meditation, tai chi, alternative healing, natural foods, etc. There was a general call to understand more about the self and each other, and tap into a broader reality. Divorce was on the rise, as people began searching for, and feeling that they had a right to, a greater sense of fulfillment from life. Life became less about survival and more about connection.

Another way to describe this transformative time is to say that it was the beginning of the transition from the Piscean Age into the Aquarian Age. Each astrological age is based on the tilt of the Earth as it spins on its axis. Each age lasts approximately 2,160 years (some resources differ on the exact number of years). Each is linked to one of the twelve astrological signs, with a full cycle beginning again every 25,920[1] years. Additionally, each age is linked to major cultural, societal and political changes on the planet.

For the last 2,100 years we were living in the Piscean Age, a time that governed the belief in hierarchical powers that lie outside of ourselves. People lived by the tenet that it was important to find someone or something externally to believe in.[2] The Piscean Age was associated with research about the truth hidden behind what is perceived by the five senses, which corresponds to the mysteries associated with Christ's life.[3] It was also the time during which the truth of our essential duality—body (form) and soul—was revealed. The evolutionary work of this Age has been the lifting of our lower physical nature to that of the soul.[4]

[1] Nicholas Campion, *The Book of World Horoscopes*, 1999, pp. 489–95.

[2] *Santokh Singh Khalsa, D.C.*, "The Aquarian Shift: What will be Different about Our World after November 11, 2011?" https://www.3ho.org/3ho-lifestyle/aquarian-age/aquarian-shift-what-will-be-different-about-our-world-after-november-11, (2011).

[3] http://en.wikipedia.org/wiki/Astrological_age#The_Age_of_Pisces_.28The_Piscean_Age.29

[4] "The Transition of the Ages Pisces to Aquarius," http://www.souledout.org/cosmology/ages/transitionages.html

Foundations of Energy Healing

The shift from the Piscean to the Aquarian Age occurred over the last fifty years. Some say the Aquarian Age began on November 11, 2011 and others say began on December 12, 2012. This new age carries with it the energy of looking within ourselves to find our power. There is an expectation that the Aquarian age will usher in a period of group consciousness.[5] As the water-bearer, Aquarius may signify that humans will be less egoistic and more in the mindset of service to others rather than service to self. We will see a rise in widespread transparent, peaceful, neighborly, and sustainable living. Humanity will evolve to understand more of its place among the stars and think more in a universal manner.[6]

The entire planet is shifting into this new vibration, this new consciousness. People are responding to the challenge of this evolution in one of two ways: either to grow more self-aware and spiritual, or to feel more fearful, angry and out of control.

The spiritual calling allows us to experience heightened senses of awareness on every level—physical, mental, emotional, and spiritual. Human beings are feeling the urge to understand themselves better, create more positive relationships and find community.

The more we get used to this new way of being with finely attuned senses and deeper connections to synchronicity and flow, we find it is the more normal way to live. Living eventually becomes being. It is a way of life devoid of the need to follow arbitrary rules, question inner guidance, and strive to achieve. Millions are waking up now; ready to heal themselves and desiring to heal others. Lightworkers everywhere are working towards

---

[5] Marcia Moore & Mark Douglas, *Astrology, The Divine Science*, Arcane Publications, York Harbour, Maine USA, 1971, Acknowledgments

[6] "The New Age of Aquarius," New-Age-of-Aquarius.com, 2012, http://www.new-age-of-aquarius.com/age-of-aquarius.html#h

"cleaning up" the impact of our fear-based beliefs in order to help life on this planet thrive—thereby creating Heaven on Earth.

This is a slow progression—a back-and-forth motion. The light and the dark are always in a dance of balance. Those that are awakening must learn to be steadfast and hold space for the positive changes that are on the way.

> *When you start to solve the problems you came (into this life with), whether it's health or relationships or life's purpose, the solutions create light. The solutions to your problems, using the creator within, creates another energy, which is light. Solution and balance create light, and this light is immediately seen by the (earth's) Crystalline Grid....Light goes into the grid and it changes the planet incrementally in a way it never did before.*
> (Kryon, Book Thirteen, The Recalibration of Humanity, p. 209.)

THE ENERGY HEALER IN THE QUANTUM FIELD

While many positive personal changes have emerged, the last sixty years has also seen an increase in maladies such as depression, suicide, rage, anxiety, stress, and addiction. As more people suffer in these ways, society looks for options to relieve their pain. More and more people are eschewing the kind of impersonal, rote western medical model that has dominated for the last one hundred years. There is a call to attend to the deeper levels of the individual with more "natural" and holistic methods of addressing the body, mind and spirit. There is a greater understanding of the fact that we are energetic beings and we can access that energy through all sorts of techniques being taught to the layperson these days, such as various forms of energy therapies, sound healing, Yoga, bodywork, psychic and astrological readings and so much more.

In the past, our notions about "healing" have been focused on fixing what was wrong. Illness was seen as the absence of wellness. The commonly held belief was that we were the victims of illness and being sick was just bad luck. Disease was seen as being caused by some invader from the outside world (bacteria, viruses, cancers) or because of some biochemical imbalance (for example, an allergy is too much histamine and depression is not enough serotonin). The goal of treatment was to kill the invader or chemically "adjust" the biochemistry by treating the symptoms.

The holistic healing model begs us to consider that physical issues may be, first, manifestations of past and present negative thoughts and emotions that form the foundation of our perceptions. Second, our perceptions create our realities. Therefore, negative thoughts and emotions (all of which stem from fear-based beliefs) attract negative experiences in our lives.

Have you awakened the healer inside yourself? Have you been healed by a holistic modality that you now want to share with others? Are you finding that you are gifted with compassion, an innate ability to move energy, or seeing deeper truths? Do you genuinely want to help people (perhaps the way you've been helped)?

The path of holistic healing through the quantum field is different from a medical model that identifies and corrects only physical ailments. In fact, healing happens in layers. The layers run through all the different lifetimes, DNA, emotional issues and soul challenges. They run through the Divine Identity, Divine Function and Divine Essence of each being, which make up the core parts of each person's personality.

No one is immune to this planet's history of violence, trauma and fear. To this end, an effective energy healer holds space for all possibilities of life. Without judgement, the energy healer enters the quantum field to remove harmful patterns from a family lineage, release trauma from this or past lifetimes, or heal the inner child.

The energy field holds patterns, the body consciousness stores cellular memory, the psyche holds emotional scars, and people create karma in their relationships. The layers of healing also run through the five energetic sheaths (or koshas), as well as

The Great Awakening

the four energy bodies: the physical, mental, emotional and spiritual bodies. (See the Chapter 3, The Human Being As Energy Being.)

We can address all this and more. And the great thing about this quantum energetic healing is that you as the healer don't need to hold all of that information, for it is a beautiful practice, replete with multitudes of angelic helpers. I call this the spiritual healing team, and they hold that knowledge of what and how to accomplish these lofty goals. This is explained in detail in Chapter 4, The Spiritual Healing Team.

Everyone alive on the planet at this time has committed to remembering themselves as aspects of Divinity, whether or not they happen to be aware of this fact. We are each choosing to do that in different ways. We each have taken different soul paths and so will have different needs during this transformation. Your job as an energy healer, or when healing yourself, is to hold space for anything that shows up, while supporting others as they remember their innate connection to Source.

Foundations of Energy Healing
ENDNOTES—CHAPTER 1

1. Nicholas Campion, *The Book of World Horoscopes*, 1999, pp. 489–95.

2. Santokh Singh Khalsa, D.C., "The Aquarian Shift: What will be Different about Our World after November 11, 2011?" www.3ho.org/3ho-lifestyle/aquarian-age/aquarian-shift-what-will-be-different-about-our-world-after-november-11, (2011).

3. en.wikipedia.org/wiki/astrological_age#The_Age_of_Pisces_.28The_Piscean_Age.29.

4. "The Transition of the Ages ⟦SEP⟧Pisces to Aquarius," www.souledout.org/cosmology/ages/transitionages.html.

5. Marcia Moore & Mark Douglas, *Astrology, The Divine Science*, Arcane Publications, York Harbour, Maine USA, 1971, Acknowledgments.

6. "The New Age of Aquarius," New-Age-of–Aquarius.com, 2012, www.new-age-of-aquarius.com/age-of-aquarius.html#h.

2. The Multi-Dimensionality of Health

What if every single cell in our bodies contained the
intelligence to function as it was designed, and also to
interact with EVERY OTHER SINGLE cell in our bodies?

We are electrical beings. We are made of energy—pure Light—and cloaked in matter that looks and feels like real, solid material. The only purpose we have here is to remember ourselves as Divine beings, sparkling extensions of our Source Creator. Our souls' missions are to remember *Who We Are*.

The soul incarnates into this body at this time to experience specific situations and challenges. Yet our experience here on this planet is only one of many aspects of our true self. We exist on many planes and many dimensions at many times simultaneously. In fact, the amount of our soul that exists within this tiny physical body is said to be less than 5 percent. That means that more than 95 percent of our Self exists beyond this particular physical manifestation. The feelings and responses to this experience are affected by the experiences and responses of all of the different aspects of our Self.

We are imprinted with memories of our experiences and our responses to them. An imprint is created by any heightened emotional response to anything that happens to us. This can be either positive or negative. For example, imagine that a young girl is getting ready for the prom. She puts on her dress and make-up and admires herself in the mirror, feeling excited or romantically dreaming of her date. Just then, her parents walked by and say, "You are the most beautiful girl. Your date is so lucky!" This would cause a positive imprint. The energy from the feelings of pride and confidence about her body and her sexuality would be held in her emotional body, and would follow her as she continued to grow up. The imprint would settle in her mental body, creating the thought that, "I am safe and confident," and her physical body would feel relaxed.

Conversely, if, while the young girl was excitedly preparing for her date, her brother comes in the room and off-handedly says, "You look stupid," it's likely that the young girl will be surprised or even shocked. That statement could surely make a lasting impression on her, causing her to feel embarrassed for primping or feeling pretty.

The energy of that would then create an imprint in her emotional body (feeling embarrassed), move into her mental body (translating into the thoughts, "I look stupid. I am ugly..." and so on), and finally settle in the physical body as, say, persistent tightness in her hips or between her shoulder blades.

In the Western medical model, when a person is not feeling well, she typically goes to a doctor who has detailed knowledge of all that is scientific and physical. One of the ways medicine shows this is through specialization, separating the parts of the body out more and more. As specialization continues to go forward, there is less recognition that all the cells in the body are affected by everything that happens in the body's energy fields, which means that every cell is connected.

In Western allopathic medicine, a doctor will diagnose and prescribe only on the basis of what hurts, what isn't functioning optimally, or what is degenerating in the body. This philosophy ignores the fact that all the parts of the body are intricately connected. And it ignores the fact that manifestations in the physical body are ultimately consequences of thoughts and emotions. I respect and honor doctors immensely, and trust me, if I were in a car accident, I would choose the ER over any place else. However, as illustrated with the young girl above, there is more than meets the eye when it comes to chronic physical issues.

The Multi-Dimensionality of Health

Likewise, when a person is depressed, anxious, or in other ways emotionally or mentally unwell, he typically seeks psychiatric care. The psychiatrist, psychologist, or social worker will talk to the person, get him to process his feelings and memories, and cognitively work through more productive ways to think and do things. I have spent years of my life in therapy, and it was very helpful in my understanding of my life and myself. However, I never felt that I fully overcame my feelings of anxiety, which seemed somehow anchored in my body.

Physical and emotional symptoms are the body's way of letting us know that there is discord in the entire system. Merely making the symptom of the discord go away does not fix the underlying problem. The body will just find another way to get our attention.

There are many alternative therapies that take more holistic approaches. I honor and respect each of these, and have used most of them myself! Each one is designed to see the person from a holistic point of view, taking into account the connection between the physical, mental, emotional and spiritual aspects of each of us. But without the full connection to the different dimensions of being and existence, complete healing cannot take place.

It has been my experience, both as a client and as a healer, that the intention of healing through a person's energy system has the potential to access multiple levels and multiple dimensions of that person, including experiences, memories, karmic patterns, and belief systems. All of this information is held in the energy that makes up the DNA, cells, muscles, bones, organs, and glands. Within this expanded perspective of healing, all aspects of an individual are addressed and people change at their core.

This quantum work has the capacity to ease depression, fatigue, anxiety, physical pain, brain fog, confusion, and fear, to name a few. It also allows for forward movement and change. All of this may be accomplished through the practices of removing the energetic imprints of trauma, clearing density and stagnation in the aura, releasing karmic ties and chords, aligning and attuning the chakras, connecting to gifts from future selves, and much, much more.

Likewise, issues that were taken on from other lifetimes may be revisited and understood in the context in which they occurred. Trauma from these lifetimes that is held in the etheric body is released. Pain in the physical body is often relieved, along with other physical issues. The being is seen as a whole—a spiritual entity moving through various experiences, all of which have an effect on the person in the present.

A DEFINITION OF *HEALING*

Healing is an internal process that restores balance and harmony to the body, mind, and spirit. Healing is a restoration of wholeness through transformation that includes growth, thereby strengthening the individual more than before the onset of dis-ease. Healing is not the mere removal or easing of symptoms, but rather an integrative process that transcends just the physical and includes all aspects of an individual.

This is different than the traditional idea of *curing*. Curing is what Western medicine attempts to do through medication, treatment, and invasive intervention. It usually is the result of a series of treatments that are designed to rid the body of the symptoms of the disease. However, in the case of chronic illness or emotional disorders, someone is completely cured only when healing happens on a deeper level.

Cancer has been cured by being cut or burned out of the body. But what healing happens in that process? Why did the cancer grow in the first place, and what was that person supposed to learn from that experience? Consider the case of someone dying from cancer: in Western medicine, doctors would say that the person has not been cured and did not heal. But suppose that, in the process of dying, the patient lovingly reconnected with family and with her personal relationship to Source. Can we surmise that those experiences of love allowed for a healing that was deeper than recovery from the illness itself?

> *As I was writing this, my kitten Fiona was in the hospital. She had been in and out of the hospital with ear infections, tumors, and irritable bowel disease for nine of the twelve months we had her. Our vet, a kind and gentle man, was trying everything to cure her. But in my discussions with my guides and Fiona herself, I understood that these were physical manifestations of millennia of traumas that Fiona was trying to clear. I became more and more certain that veterinary assistance was not going to be helpful other than to make her, when possible, more comfortable. Fiona was intent on healing her issues in this lifetime, and, while there were indeed medicines that could help her feel better and dissipate the infections, there was no cure for her release of karmic patterns.*

THE HEALER DEFINED

The healer is the facilitator and conduit for healing to happen. Everyone brings her own skills and gifts to this process. Please do not get caught up in only the traditional idea of a medicine man or Indian shaman, or an extreme religious healer who sends people into ecstatic experiences, or even the crystal-carrying, "WooWoo" New Age healer. Anyone who has the desire can be the person who holds space, sets the intention to facilitate change, connects to the quantum field, and enables the magic of transformation to happen.

Do you need a practitioner to do this for you? Not necessarily. All people have access to their own guides and healing team, and in setting the intention to heal or shift or change, they begin to do so. But the subconscious mind keeps wounds and traumas safely hidden from view, so it is not necessarily possible for human beings to uncover their own issues. It often takes another person to help to identify or access that information.

The power of two people's intentions is greater than the sum of both. And the four points—the healer, client, guides, and healing team—is a stronger structure than three points that is created between the client, the guide, and the healing team. Think of a table with four legs versus one with three.

I have found for myself, and seen in numerous clients, quantum energy healing results in more complete change, with longer-lasting effects. I have experienced for myself, and seen in these clients, quick shifts into calmer, more peaceful, more productive life choices.

HOW DOES THIS HAPPEN?

We are all co-creators of our lives and everything that exists on this planet. We create our experiences through our beliefs, both personally and en masse. Quantum physics has proven that belief in what we expect to see shapes what is going to happen. Intention creates results.

When I first became a Reiki healer, my teacher told me that I would begin to sense guides and healers working with me. I was eager for this experience, and by the time I was a Reiki Level 2, I could feel others in my presence while I was healing. When I became Reiki Level 3, in accordance with my expectations, I began to see the guides, and their presence was ever more real. My hands would become someone else's hands. I could see in my mind's eye what to do ahead of time. While my hands were in one place, I could see other beings working on my clients in other areas of their bodies.

Personally, I never questioned this. During the sessions, it was clear that I had assistance, although after the fact, I often shook my head in disbelief and wondered if I wasn't losing my mind.

The Multi-Dimensionality of Health

For me, sessions are always hazy afterwards, as there is a kind of built-in amnesia effect when working in the other dimensional planes. A great many healers and channelers I know have told me they feel they might be crazy. I assure them that we all feel this way. What seems natural and obvious while in an altered state seems unbelievable and implausible in the conscious state.

It is also my belief that every healer—whether a doctor, psychiatrist, psychologist, massage therapist, or other healer—has a spiritual healing team. I believe this because I know that these higher-energy beings LOVE us and are committed to service for our well-being and spiritual growth. It is my belief that all beings on the planet has this kind of support, whether they are aware of it or not.

Guides and angels are dedicated to helping us all achieve our goals.

I have deemed this support group the *spiritual healing team*, consisting of angels, archangels, ascended masters, elohim, ETs, and other members of the Collective. Each of these beings is dedicated to assisting us with our ascension by clearing past traumas, soothing our emotional systems, and preparing our energy fields for increased access to the Light. It may feel important to you to begin to discern who is with you, and you can do this by simply asking, or having another intuitive person help you. The following chapters will go into much more detail about this.

Knowing this and setting the intention to use these Light-beings in our healing sessions adds to their power. We become the conscious conduit for their energies. It is at this point that we must move beyond the ego state of thinking we know what to do, and into the position of facilitator for much greater work that is being done. A conduit holds, directs, and organizes the intense energies coming in from the Lightbeings. Doing this focuses the energies of the Lightbeings by creating a channel through which they can direct their healing intelligence.

15

Foundations of Energy Healing

Included in the spiritual healing team are also the client's *spirit guides*. The client's guides know all aspects of the person and assess what is for her highest good at any given time. They know the soul's ultimate goals. In that way, the guides direct the flow of what needs to be released and healed, and which issues are still in process—allowing for certain circumstances that are ultimately serving the soul's purpose. They operate in complete and utter LOVE and support the person through the release of pain and suffering, while finding the best outcomes for the highest good of all involved.

The client's guides are the true directors of the healing process. They run the show. The spiritual healing team shows up based on that, and the healer facilitates the process on the physical level. I will explain in greater detail how to deepen your awareness of this process in further chapters, while also incorporating your skills and expertise to make each session uniquely yours.

3. The Human Being as Energy Being

*What if our boundaries extended far beyond those
of the physical body that we feel and experience
with our usual senses?*

Human beings are comprised of a vast and complicated energy system that moves from the highest vibration in the outermost fields, to the densest vibration, which is the physical matter that comprises the human body. Many people think that the physical body is the primary body and all the other energy bodies emanate from it. However, the opposite is actually true: the physical body resides inside the energy bodies.

There is a grid of energy that holds the whole system "together." It is a vast web of interlocking geometries whose lines connect the various bodies and the blueprint for the physical body. This Flower of Life is a sacred geometry consisting of interlocking circles. Triangles connect all the energy points in and around the body, and within each chakra as well. Each triangle is a facet of our personalities.

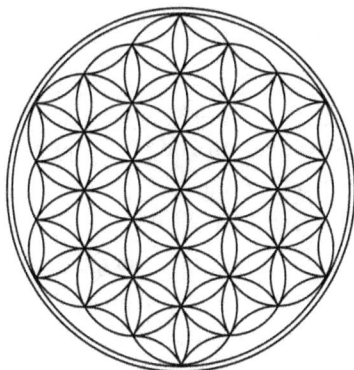

This grid also connects the human system to the planet's own grid, which in turn is connected to every other animal, vegetable and mineral. In truth, there is NO energetic separation from anything or anyone on this planet.

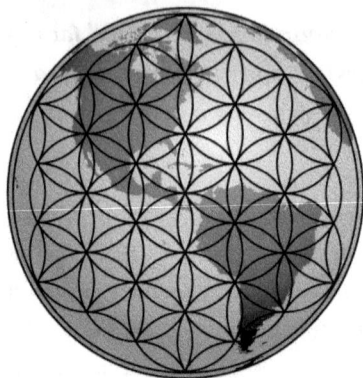

Aspects of us exist on multiple dimensions at the same time. Each soul's particular energy system is connected to its Oversoul (Higher Self), and to the Lightbeings—the ascended masters, angels, archangels, elohim, seraphim, alien races—and, finally, God, the Source of All That Is. Again, there is no actual separation of any of us. There is only the personality of each human being that exists in a separate body in an effort to create the experience of individuality.

The electromagnetic field of energy surrounding our physical bodies is broken down into the etheric body (or the aura), the emotional body, the mental body and the spiritual body. This energy field is both a transmitter and a receiver, reaching out to and responding to others on the planet at all times. It keeps us connected and it *is* our connection. As our energy fields overlap with other people's, with that of the animals, trees, rocks and the Earth herself, we truly are All One coinciding field of energy, and we constantly move in and out of resonance with others. This makes us walking, talking barometers of thoughts, feelings and emotions, constantly registering those of ourselves and everyone and everything around us.

This kind of connection shows up in a myriad of ways. For instance, many people feel uneasy when there is any kind of unrest halfway across the world. I know people (myself included) that are intensely connected to weather changes before they happen. And there are also many people who dream of world events right before they occur.

These are only some of the ways these energy bodies feed knowledge to us, potentially causing us to have seemingly rational or irrational thoughts, emotions and feelings. When we are out of balance, we may identify with one body more than the other. For instance, a person may be "all in his head," meaning that he is identifying with his mental body, and thus deems cognition and rational thought to be more important than his emotions or physical feelings. Alternatively, a person may allow his emotions to rule, disregarding rational thought processes or physical sensations.

Each energy body informs—and ultimately forms—the physical body. Negative thoughts, beliefs and emotions stem from fear. The prevalent illusion of disconnection from Source perpetuates beliefs in lack, scarcity, worry, control, loneliness, confusion, doubt, distrust... all aspects of fear. Eventually, these feelings have negative impacts on the physical body, creating dis-ease—illness, pain, and other physical suffering. These are the body's way of signaling to us that we are having false thoughts and beliefs.

The ultimate goal is to bring all of these important information systems held in the energy bodies into balance, utilizing the wisdom of each. The spiritual body can offer information from the soul and Divine connection, the mental body can offer helpful thoughts about experiences and new facts, the emotional body can support these with positive feelings devoid of fear, and the physical body can move us through our physical experiences with ease, grace and joy.

Foundations of Energy Healing

THE SPIRITUAL BODY

The spiritual body is the finest vibration and is the bridge between our conscience and our consciousness. It is the energy field that connects us to our Higher Selves, Soul, Soul Group, and ultimately, Source. It can be difficult to receive clear communication from these higher aspects of self when any of the other bodies are out of balance.

When stuck in the illusion of separation from Source, we are at risk of ignoring messages brought in through the spiritual body. Thus, when these messages hit the mental body, there is the potential to believe they are not real. When the messages hit the emotional body, there is the potential to shut them down.

However, if we are balanced in our receptivity of these intricate information systems, life flows to us. Opportunities appear and synchronies happen. Also, when we receive messages from Source enter our fields, we are able to acknowledge and follow them without hesitation. No longer do we think, "I must be crazy," or "Why is this happening?" Instead, it becomes automatic to accept that we are more than the body, fully connected to a greater Source that is guiding us and supporting us to follow our paths with ease, and we oblige.

THE MENTAL BODY

The mental body is the home of the intellect and operates at a higher frequency than the emotional body. It houses the mind. The mind is not in the brain. The mind surrounds the entire body.

Long-held and repetitive thoughts can turn into *thoughtforms*, thoughts that actually become physical clouds of matter. These are somewhat more difficult to remove or change, but is it far from impossible. We are all capable of mastering our thoughts and creating new belief systems. The easiest way to do this is to recognize the discomfort we feel when a false thought arises. (The discomfort is the signal that this is a false thought.) Choose a more positive, divinely connected thought and mentally and visually place the new thought on top of the old one.

Here is a quick Neuro-Linguistic Programing (NLP) technique to reframe a false thought and its resulting feeling, using as an example, "I don't have enough money." This thought may make me feel depressed or scared, and it may give me a stomach ache. And moving my awareness into my body, I can visualize this conglomeration of feelings as a sickly green color.

I quickly decide that this thought is disconnected from my true Self, which is divinely connected to Source. To change my thinking, I come up with the new affirmation, "God and the Universe provide for me everything that I need." This new positive thought allows me to feel hopeful and lighter in my body. I can visualize this feeling as a light yellow color.

Closing my eyes, I place this light yellow "swatch" of color on top of the sickly green, covering it completely. Light yellow now influences and becomes my governing thought and feeling. In the beginning of this process, I may have to do this 50 times a day, then 30 times a day, then 10 times a day. But eventually, if I stick to it, the new positive belief replaces the old negative one.

The reason this is important to understand is because our thoughts are creative. This Earth-bound reality is a big reflecting pool and what we put out there is what we get back. Our repeated negative thoughts are the forces behind unwelcome outcomes.

The Universe does not know whether the vibration that you're offering is because of something you're observing or something you're remembering or something that you are imagining. It just receives the vibration and answers it with things that match it.

—ABRAHAM-HICKS, EXCERPTED FROM NAPA, CA ON 2/27/1997

THE EMOTIONAL BODY

The emotional body is normally about two to six feet beyond the body's physical surface perimeter, but it can be much larger in some people. This is literally where your emotions reside. It is also where you pick up other people's emotions. It is important to know which emotions you are generating yourself versus which you are detecting in other people. Remember that you have control over the energy you allow in your emotional field.

Many people know themselves to be empaths, those who pick up the feelings of others. A good example of this is when you go to a party and you can pick out the person in the room who is feeling left out, without knowing anything about that person. Another example is when you are in a public place, like a restaurant, and another customer walks by you and you suddenly become uneasy.

In truth, we are all empathic, but some are more sensitive ones… and therefore potentially more uncomfortable because of it. Be conscious of how your feelings change to learn how to discern between whose feelings are whose, and to rid yourself of others' emotions that are unnecessary. The easiest way to do this when suddenly experiencing an emotion that feels extreme, or one that does not make sense to you, is to simply ask, "Who does this belong to?" If the feeling moves away or becomes lighter, it is not yours. State, "Back to sender!" You will feel a sense of relief.

THE ETHERIC BODY AND THE MERIDIANS

The etheric body is the energy field immediately surrounding your body—about a half-inch off your physical body. The etheric body holds the karmic patterns of the personality and the physicality, called the etheric blueprint, and it exists on many dimensions at once, from the fourth through the seventh.

The Human Being as Energy Being

Acupuncture meridians exist within the fourth dimension and the etheric body is formed around them. Meridians are the energetic channels through which life force energy (called *chi* in Traditional Chinese Medicine and *prana* in Ayurvedic Medicine) flows. Our physical health is dependent on the vitality of the flow of energies through the meridians.

The meridian system is complex, explained through five elements and twelve major meridians. Following is a very brief description of a system that normally takes volumes to explain in detail.

The five elements, which are reflected in the macrocosm of nature, as well as in the microcosm of our bodies and personalities, include: Wood, Fire, Earth, Air and Water. Each element governs two meridians, except the Fire element, which controls four.

The twelve meridians are: Liver, Gallbladder, Heart, Heart Protector, Small Intestine, Triple Burner, Stomach, Spleen, Lung, Large Intestine, Kidney and Bladder. (Two other meridians, the Conception Vessel and the Governing Vessel, are not tied to the elements.) In Chinese medicine, the meridians are given jobs and duties, as if they were twelve officials governing a kingdom. Each official rules specific physiological functions, organs and parts of the body, as well as emotional and psychological functions.

The Wood element is comprised of the Liver and Gallbladder meridians. These meridians govern the season of Spring, a time of dynamic growth and activity. Accordingly, they are responsible for initiating change, guiding our development and granting us our ability to mature. They give us the ability to assert who we are to the rest of the world.

The Wood element governs the emotion of anger, as well as its opposite, being unassertive and unwilling to provoke any situation that might produce conflict. At times, we all "lose our way," discovering ourselves in situations where creativity and assertive aspects cannot find expression. Our lives stagnate rather than evolve in response to our own changing needs. Frustration, irritability, resentment and despondency are common results.

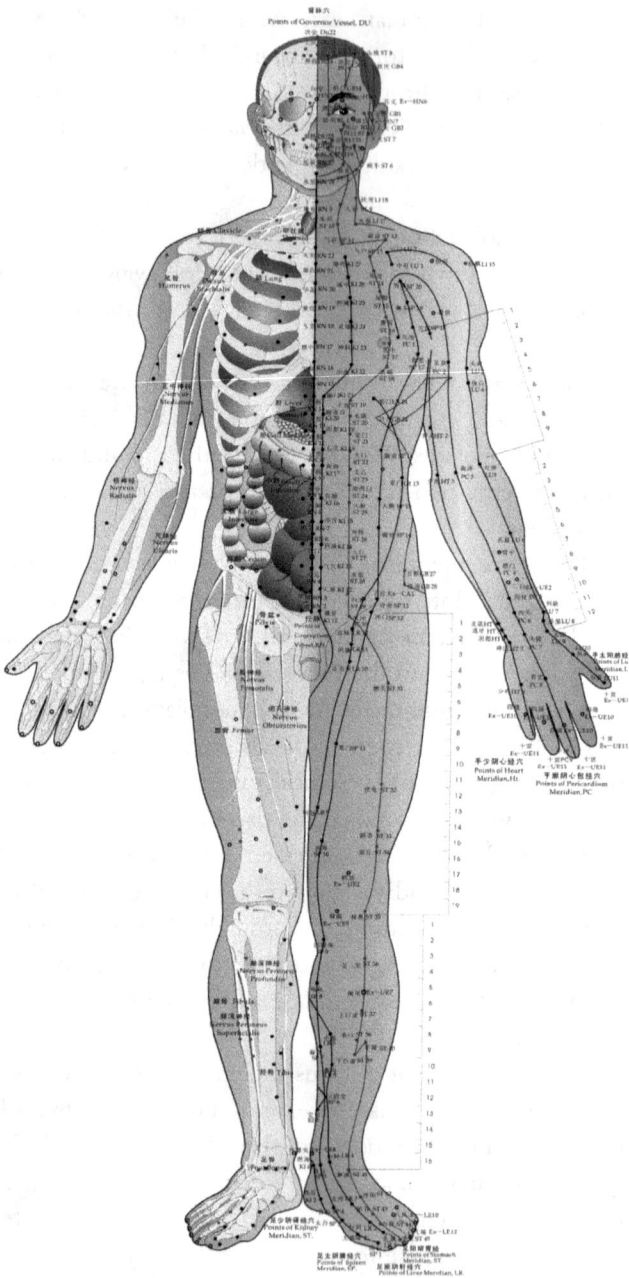

The meridian system—front

The Human Being as Energy Being

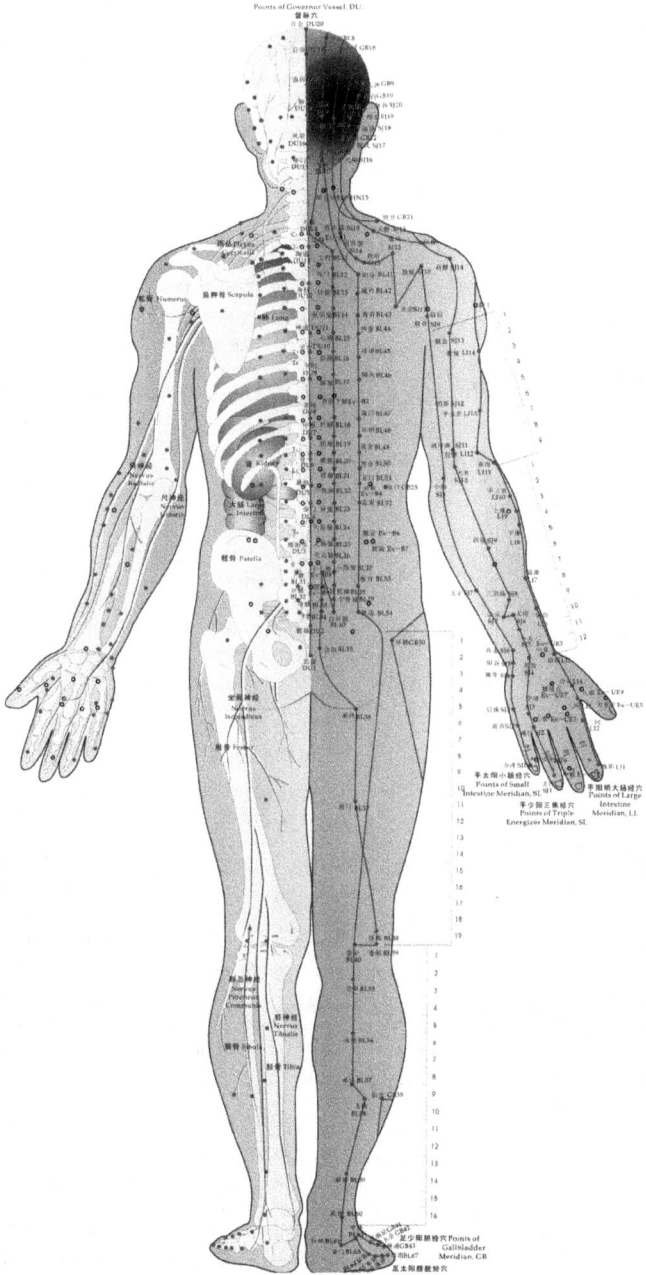

The meridian system—back

25

Opening the flow of energy through the Liver and Gallbladder meridians can remedy this.

The Fire element is comprised of four meridians: the Heart, Heart Protector, Small Intestines and Triple Burner. This element governs the season of Summer. It is responsible for the qualities we draw upon to relate to and bond with other people. Through these meridians, we can affect feelings of loneliness and a longing for intimacy, as well as feelings of rejection or being unwanted. As we create flow throughout these energy centers we enable ourselves to experience sparkle, joy and warmth.

The Earth element is comprised of the Stomach and Spleen meridians. Its season is late summer. These meridians are responsible for giving stability and the ability to adjust to differing circumstances and to cope with difficulties. Dysfunctional energy flow through these meridians manifests as worry, preoccupation and obsessional thoughts and behaviors. The type of person with this issue looks to others for sympathy and support.

The Stomach and Spleen meridians are also linked to nourishment of the mind, body and spirit. This is related to food, home, travel and our relationship with our mothers.

The Metal element is comprised of the Lung and Large Intestine meridians. This element governs autumn, a time of decline when nature draws into itself. Therefore, metal governs feelings of grief, sadness, melancholy, disappointment and regret.

When life loses its richness, cynicism, boredom and apathy may be experienced, as well as self-doubt and lack of self-worth. Balancing the flow of energy through the Lung and Large Intestine meridians help to revive a sense of richness and quality to one's inner life. These meridians also govern our relationship with our father and father-figures.

The Water element is comprised of the Kidney and Bladder meridians. This element governs the season of winter. This element is the most difficult to perceive, yet is the foundation for all the other energies. It is the origin of our congenital "essence" (*Jing*) which determines our basic constitution and our ability to develop through the stages of growth. Imbalances in these meridians create the sense of fear, anxiety, suspicion and paranoia. However, when Water is healthy, a person is emotionally balanced and constitutionally strong.

It is helpful to have at least a basic understanding of where these meridians exist in the body, as it is likely that there will be times when you will run energy into specific points on your client's body. It can be useful to understand which meridian you are accessing, as this gives you information into the emotional and physiological issues of their bodies.

THE ETHERIC CIRCULATORY SYSTEM

The fifth-dimensional etheric blueprint is made up of another, different meridian and circulatory system, as well as spin points through which these systems and structures are connected. Fifth-dimensional meridians are the equivalent of acupuncture meridians, but they connect us with our Oversouls and Source Creator. They are the lines of energy that tether our spirits to our bodies, and our bodies to Source. This is one description of how this works:

> *Picture the Milky Way as the body of a living conscious being. The stars and planets are organs in the body; all the different species on the stars and planets are like cells in the organs of the collective body, renewing the energies of the organs and cells. Planet Earth and her inhabitants were separated from the galactic body and the Oversoul to play this game of separation, and are now being reconnected (through these fifth-dimensional meridians).*[1]

The meridian lines within the etheric circulatory system are made of Light and Sound. They lie along the acupuncture meridians and connect into some of them by means of "spin points." Spin points are small spherical vortexes of electromagnetic energy that feel like they are on the surface of the skin. (There are also spin points in every cell of the body.) These cellular points emit Sound and Light frequencies that spin the atoms of the molecules in the cell at a faster rate. Through the increased molecular speed, Light fibers are created that set up a grid for cellular regeneration.

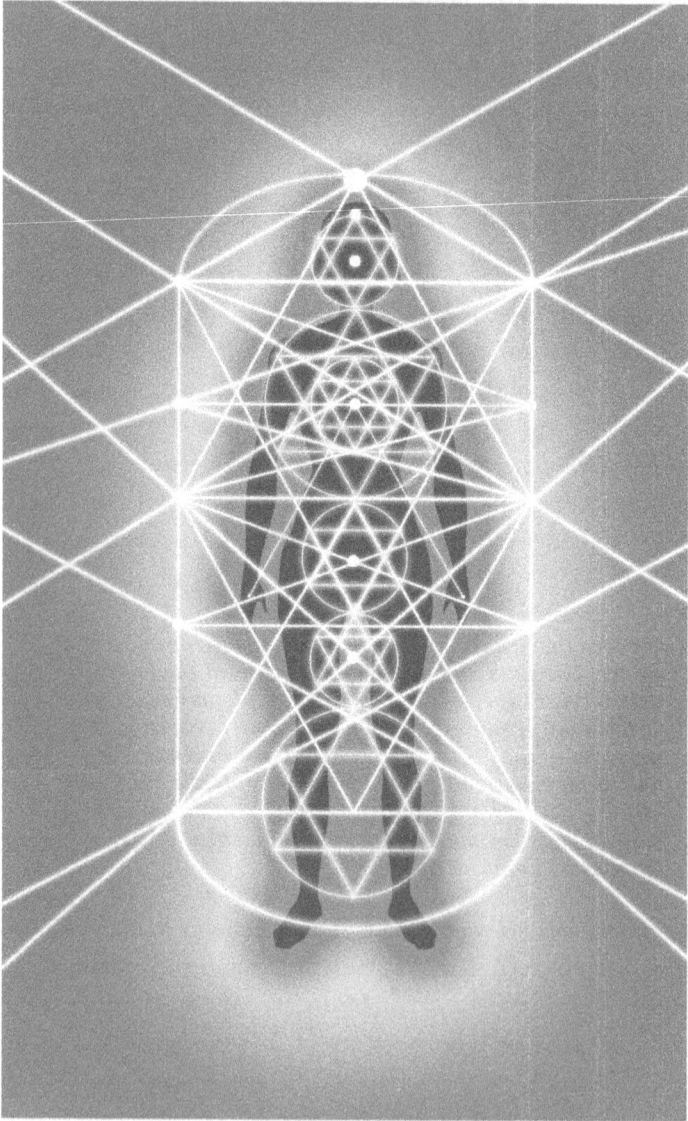

The etheric circulatory system.

The etheric circulatory system's meridians connect the spin points on the skin's surface to every spin point in every cell. This "axial system" pulses energy like the circulatory system pulses the blood, but is basically electrical in nature, like the nervous system. The Oversoul sends energy into the axiotonal lines, which then goes into the spin points on the surface of the skin, feeding the physical acupuncture meridians and then the axial system. As it does so, it wakes the human system up, creating perfect health and, ultimately, mankind's ascension. In so doing, these energy points create a model for physical transmutation.[2]

THE 14 CHAKRAS

The chakras are wheels of energy existing at intersections along the body's energy grid. They are frequency transformers for energy, connectors of the energy that flows into our fields from the external environment. This influx of external information mixes with our experiences and our belief systems. This process creates our perceptions of reality.

EXPERIENCES + BELIEF SYSTEMS = PERCEPTIONS OF REALITY

Prior to incarnation, our souls agree to certain life issues. These are created through constrictions that are imprinted in the chakras, activated at pre-appointed moments, and made manifest in our bodies and lives as challenges that demand attention. Money issues, relationships, family dysfunction, illness and more are pre-programmed into the chakra energy centers. As we embrace them as opportunities for growth instead of as experiences of victimization and powerlessness, their transformation provides the fuel for our spiritual evolution.[3] Look for the behavior patterns that repeat themselves, for these are the indications of these spiritual life lessons.

Foundations of Energy Healing

There are seven major chakras, located vertically along the spine, that have the greatest significance. They are listed below. There are also secondary chakras at the spleen and thymus, which are mentioned in many healing modalities. Additionally, there are minor chakras at every joint in the body, the hands and the feet.

Each chakra resides in the etheric body and moves energy into the physical body. They are normally described as cone-shaped, wider farther away from the physical body, and narrower closer to the center of the body. They radiate both from the front and back of the body.

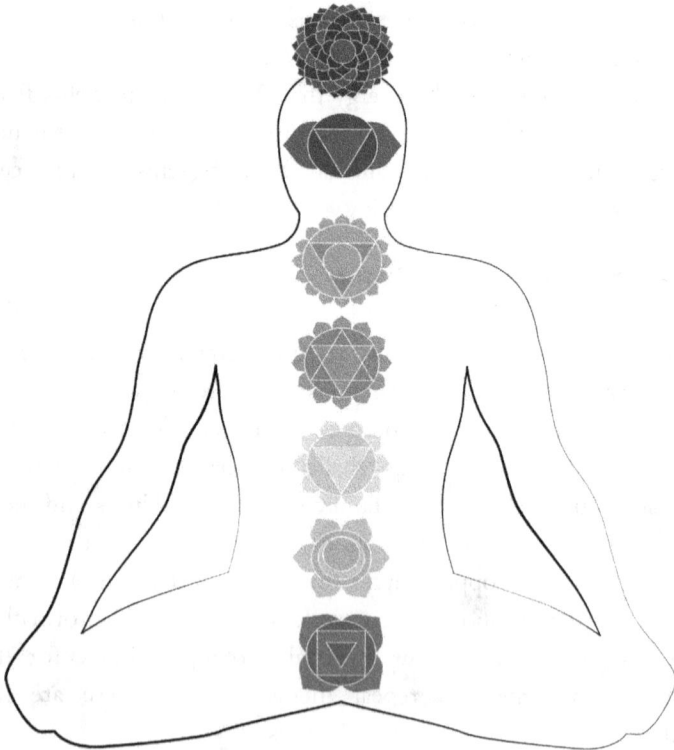

The seven major chakras.

The Human Being as Energy Being

The energies coming in from the front of the chakras are related to *manifestation*. "The energies entering from the back of the chakras are related to *will*. The rear of the chakra holds potential for action that the front of the chakra…can use as needed for its creating, its vitality of the (grid), and its interaction with the world."[4]

The reason for the cone shape is that within third-dimensional reality the chakras have been limited, and thus, "sealed" in order to perpetuate the illusion of separation.

The narrow part in the middle tends to be clogged with emotional "debris," causing the spin of the cones to slow down or stop. This starves the acupuncture meridian system of energy and can cause illness or death. This type of chakra structure can only move energy front to back or back to front, and cannot utilize higher-dimensional frequencies.[5]

OVERVIEW OF THE CHAKRAS

Chakra:	One
Name:	Root or Base
Location:	Base of spine
Element:	Earth
Color:	Red
Gland:	Reproductive glands
Manifestation:	To be here, to have
Will:	Survival, personality
Emotion:	Bravery
Goals:	Safety, stability, grounding, prosperity, right livelihood, financial abundance
Malfunction:	Obesity, hemorrhoids, constipation, frequent illness, fears, spaciness
Other associated body parts:	Legs, feet, bones, large intestine, nose

Foundations of Energy Healing

Chakra:	Two
Name:	Naval / Sacral
Location:	Lower abdomen
Element:	Water
Color:	Orange
Gland:	Adrenal glands
Manifestation:	To feel, to want
Will:	Passion, raw emotions
Emotion:	Creativity
Goals:	Emotional fluidity, pleasure, relaxation, creativity, nurturance
Malfunction:	Sexual dysfunction, isolation, emotional instability, bladder problems, numbness
Other associated body parts:	Sex organs, bladder, kidneys, tongue

Chakra:	Three
Name:	Solar plexus
Location:	Solar plexus
Element:	Fire
Color:	Yellow
Gland:	Pancreas
Manifestation:	Discernment, boundaries
Will:	Motivation
Emotion:	Laughter, anger, joy
Goals:	Vitality, healthy ego strength, purpose, integrity, structure, self-esteem
Malfunction:	Ulcers, diabetes, hypoglycemia, timidity, dominant, digestive problems
Other associated body parts:	Musculature, digestive organs

Chakra:	Four
Name:	Heart
Location:	Heart center
Element:	Air
Color:	Green, pink
Gland:	Thymus
Manifestation:	To love and be loved
Will:	Protection, preparation to give to self and others
Emotion:	Compassion
Goals:	Acceptance, forgiveness, joy, trust, vulnerability, fear of being hurt
Malfunction:	Asthma, heart problems, loneliness, co-dependence, resentment, bitterness
Other associated body parts:	Lungs, heart, breasts, arms, hands, skin

Chakra:	Five
Name:	Throat
Location:	Throat
Element:	Ether and sound
Color:	Bright blue
Gland:	Thyroid
Manifestation:	Worthiness
Will:	Integrity
Emotion:	Creative expression
Goals:	Gratitude, beliefs about abundance, speaking the truth, communication
Malfunction:	Thyroid, sore throat, neck ache, poor communication, holding back truth, addiction, shame
Other associated body parts:	Throat, mouth, ears, arms, hands

Overview of the Chakras (cont.)

Chakra:	Six
Name:	Brow
Location:	Third eye
Element:	Light
Color:	Indigo blue
Gland:	Pituitary
Manifestation:	Power of sight and thought
Will:	Intuition, true sight
Emotion:	Creative imagination
Goals:	Insight, psychic perception, divine memory, wonder
Malfunction:	Headaches, nightmares, hallucinations, blindness, preconceived notions, pride
Other associated body parts:	Eyes

Chakra:	Seven
Name:	Crown
Location:	Top of head
Element:	Thought
Color:	Violet or white
Gland:	Pineal
Manifestation:	To know
Will:	Clarity, doubt
Emotion:	Bliss
Goals:	Wisdom, knowledge, spiritual connection, selflessness, oneness
Malfunction:	Neurological disorders, depression, apathy, alienation, confusion, overly intellectual
Other associated body parts:	Cerebral cortex

It is said that over time, as our vibrations rise and we move through the ascension process, theses seals will be broken. Then the chakras will become spherical in shape, radiating energies from all directions. The body will shed its karmic debris and the spheres will expand in size until they all merge at the heart, creating one unified heart chakra. All of our motivation will emanate from the heart.

From a spiritual perspective, the chakras allow us to co-create both with Source and our Souls, and therefore actualize and manifest on this planet, all the while moving through the ascension process. From the higher chakras down, we draw on our Soul energies to manifest our desires (whether they are conscious or unconscious desires):

- The 7th Chakra (crown) is our connection to *inspiration*, the thought before the thought.

- The 6th chakra (brow) brings into consciousness the *idea*, the manifestation of inspiration.

- The 5th chakra (throat) allows us to *verbalize* and *communicate* an idea, both to ourselves and to others.

- The 4th chakra (heart) moves the idea from the *spiritual* perspective to the *Earthly* perspective, where we ask ourselves if we feel safe enough to bring it through.

- The 3rd chakra (solar plexus) gives us the *drive* to begin to manifest an idea into matter.

- The 2nd chakra (sacrum) stores our *creativity* and *fertility*, bringing life to our creations.

- And the 1st chakra (base) is the creation of *matter* on the planet.

At the same time, human beings are moving *up* through the ascension process continually, on a global scale, as well as on the personal scale, throughout lifetimes, as well as on the level of individual experiences. This is illustrated through the energies of the chakras, from the first to the seventh:

- The 1st chakra governs our survival issues.

- The 2nd chakra governs our relationship issues.

- The 3rd chakra governs our sense of personal power and integrity. The three together are said to regulate our energies for being earthbound.

- The 4th chakra, with its energies of unconditional love and forgiveness, bridge the lower three and upper three chakras.

- Continuing up the ladder of ascension, the 5th chakra controls the energies for our wills and our gratitude.

- The 6th chakra allows us to connect to our intuition and greater knowing.

- And, finally, the 7th chakra is our connection to Spirit, to Ultimate Wisdom. These three upper chakras regulate our spiritual energies.

The key to self-mastery is living with all seven chakras being open, in alignment and spinning in unison—vibrating with the safety and knowledge that we are each an aspect of God having a physical experience in a world of free will.

Additionally, some authors write that there are seven more, higher chakras. The first three of these are connected to the energy bodies, and the upper four are connected to aspects of the soul. I have seen this described by numerous sources as follows:

- 8th chakra – the Emotional body

- 9th chakra – the Mental body

- 10th chakra – the Spiritual body

- 11th chakra – the Oversoul

- 12th chakra – Christ Oversoul

- 13th chakra – I Am Oversoul

- 14th chakra – Keter Oversoul (*Keter* is Hebrew for *crown*)

In his book *Soul Psychology*, Joshua David Stone writes that there are 22 chakras, numbers 8 through 15 exist in the 4th dimension, and 16 through 22 exist in the fifth dimension. I have not seen that information elsewhere. These fifth-dimensional chakras connect us to ascension, universal light, divine intent, universal energy, beingness, divine structure, and Source, respectively. (Practice the Chakra Balance meditation in Chapter 9, Mind-Body Practices, or listen to the recording online at randibotnick.com/listeninglibrary.)

THE PHYSICAL BODY AND THE FIVE KOSHAS

How does the illusion of separation result in the energy blockages that actually forms physical illness? One of the earliest models of this concept is described in the Vedic tradition's *Taittiriya Upanishad*, dating from around 800 BC. It describes five sheaths, called the five *koshas*, comprising the human being. A sheath is defined as a close-fitting case or covering. The five sheaths, or koshas, exist within the body. The level of harmony within the energy flow among these layers determines the health and well-being of the individual.

The five koshas are each made of increasingly more and more subtle energy. The idea behind separating these sheaths is to show the Unity that manifests in different forms in each of our lives. Understanding and developing our koshas help us to grow spiritually. As you read below, you will notice that they are described like a mirror image of the energy bodies.

It is written in the *Taittiriya Upanishad*:

Foundations of Energy Healing

Human beings consist of a material body built from the food they eat. Those who care for this body are nourished by the universe itself.

Inside this is another body made of life energy. It fills the physical body and takes its shape. Those who treat this vital force as divine experience excellent health and longevity because this energy is the source of physical life.

Within the vital force is yet another body, this one made of thought energy. It fills the two denser bodies and has the same shape. Those who understand and control the mental body are no longer afflicted by fear.

Deeper still lies another body comprised of intellect. It permeates the three denser bodies and assumes the same form. Those who establish their awareness here free themselves from unhealthy thoughts and actions, and develop the self-control necessary to achieve their goals.

Hidden inside it is yet a subtler body, composed of pure joy. It pervades the other bodies and shares the same shape. It is experienced as happiness, delight, and bliss.

The first kosha is the physical body (in Sanskrit called the *annamaya kosha*), the material one with which we most easily identify. All the different body systems are contained within this sheath.[6]

The second kosha (called the *pranamaya kosha*) consists of *prana*, meaning life force energy. Prana is like an organizing field that gives life to the physical body. Stress and nervous tension lead to blockages in the flow of breath, which is thought to be the foundation of health at all levels. However, this sheath is replenished through breathing practices (in yoga, *pranayama* is the practice of the breath), eating healthy, whole foods, and getting plenty of sunlight (the ultimate source of prana).

The third kosha (the *manomaya kosha*) is called the mental body, what we may call body consciousness or the subconscious mind. With its own life force, the nervous system controls this kosha. This is the automatic pilot that exists within us, pumping our heart, moving our blood, digesting our food, without any thought or control from our minds. Angry and violent thoughts and images distress and disrupt the mental body, while practices such as meditation and hypnosis support and nourish it.

The fourth kosha (the *jnanamaya kosha*) is often translated as "intellect," and it comprises our conscience, will power, and ethics. It is said that with a poorly developed intellect body, people live lives that feel out of control, where they are always in a state of reaction to chaotic situations. People with a poorly developed fourth kosha may live double lives, espousing one set of moral doctrines, but privately engaging in unethical scenarios. Life may be seen as unfair, competitive, and difficult. There is a whole practice of yoga, called *Jnana yoga* (translated as "the yoga of knowledge"), that helps create a healthy fourth kosha through contemplation and incorporation of spiritual truths.

And finally, the fifth kosha (the *anandamaya kosha*) is the bliss body, and it is the thinnest veil that stands between our ordinary awareness and our higher Self. In a meditation practice, you might hear it referred to as the brilliant white light in the center of your being. This kosha is disturbed and unbalanced when people feel that they are alone in the world. This sets off a whole series of beliefs, psychological processes, energetic blockages, and physical symptoms that detract from our natural state of bliss and happiness.[7] However, the yoga tradition says this body is awakened and strengthened through the practices of selfless service, devotion to God and heart-opening meditations. (Practice the Experiencing Your Five Koshas meditation in Chapter 9, Mind-Body Practices, or listen to the recording online at randibot-nick.com/listeninglibrary.)

■ ■ ■ ■ ■ ■ ■

I cannot stress enough how important it is to understand the human energy field that reaches deep inside the physical body and well out beyond it, ultimately, infinitely. Understanding all of the bodies that comprise a human being provides us with a vast picture of the truth of Who We Are. The movement of information throughout this system is constant. Our experiences and beliefs begin in and reside in these fields, and are the source of all health and wellness as well as all dis-ease and illness.

The vast system that comprises the energy bodies, chakras, and koshas paints the picture of us as dynamic beings experiencing a reality that is far smaller than our true nature. We are, indeed, spiritual beings having human experiences. On a grand scale, we are connected to everything and everyone. We can open our minds to communicate with the rest of the Universe, whether

---

HOME PRACTICE

Practice the Body Awareness Exercise included in Chapter 10, Mind-Body Practices. A recording of this guided meditation may also be found online at randibotnick.com/listeninglibrary.

This Body Awareness Exercise brings you into intimate contact with your physical self. As you watch your breath, you can begin to see the quality of the energy within and around your body. You may even notice the chakras and the aura. Or you may experience your body merge with the energy around you. The possibilities are limitless.

ENDNOTES: CHAPTER 3

1. Tashira Tachi-ren, *What is Lightbody?* (1999, Lithia Springs, GA: World Tree Press.) p. 30.

2. Ibid. p. 31.

3. Jonathan M. Goldman, M.Ac., *Gift of the Body: A MultiDimensional Guide to Energy Anatomy, Grounded Spirituality and Living Through the Heart.* (2014, Bend, OR: Essential Light Institute.) p. 132.

4. Ibid. p. 113.

5. Tashira Tachi-ren, p. 33.

6. Joseph LePage, *Integrative Yoga Therapy Manual* (1994), p. 21.

7. Ibid. p. 2.3.

4. The Spiritual Healing Team

What if the room we were in right now was filled with
beings, beyond detection by our usual senses,
waiting for an invitation to help us?

As we open into quantum energy healing, awareness moves between the feeling that the healing is *apart from* us and the feeling that it is *a part of* us. Indeed, both are true in that we are tapping into the cosmic consciousness in which we are connected to the all-knowing, all-loving, all-powerful, universal life-force energies. At the same time, spiritual beings come to assist us with the process.

The great Madame Blavatsky, a renowned channel and psychic who lived from 1831 to 1891, was one of the founders of the Theosophical Society and author of many books of channeled information. Madame Blavatsky credited the ascended masters for much of her supernatural abilities, of which there were many. She reportedly could materialize objects out of thin air, receive precise written information before her in "astral light," and spontaneously create masterful works of art. And while she channeled and taught the words of the masters, the masters themselves were later to say that she created many of the supernatural miracles that she performed alone, without their help.[1]

There is no more time to stand in our ego-driven beliefs that we are alone on this planet, forsaken with only this one lifetime and this one dimension. On the contrary, we have an infinite supply of help and Love and Light to call on. Lightbeings are here now, just waiting for us to ask for their assistance. A plethora of beings have been called on from all corners of the Universe to assist us in our awakening through healing, love, wisdom, guidance, and more. They want nothing more than for us to remember our power in the process of our co-creation of heaven on Earth. In fact, our ascension aids them in theirs.

Just as we have incarnated in these physical bodies, and we are taking part in an existence that permits us to experience ourselves individually, spiritual beings also individuate and express themselves through us to assist us in whatever we do. These beings are often called guardian angels, guides, archangels, and ascended masters. The unseen world is vast and infinite. There are countless numbers of individuated spirits that come to help us. I am sure many are still beyond our comprehension.

I have termed this group of beings who joins us in the healing sessions as the *spiritual healing team*, and I have worked with all the divine beings listed below at one point or another. You may do the same, or you may be someone who is linked to one particular group only. I know healers who work primarily with Archangel Michael or Saint Germain, for example, and don't have (conscious) relationships with others. As I say throughout this book, each healer is unique. You may find it helpful and comforting to identify who is included in your spiritual healing team.

Invite in individual entities whenever you feel called to. They are all-loving, nonjudgmental beings, who first and foremost respect our free will, so they do not intervene unless invited. However, once you open the door, they know they are welcome. So before you begin your healing practice, you may wish to connect with your guides and state your intentions. For example:

> *I am open to all healing energies that are of the Light. I draw to me all those who wish to help me, and any of my clients, on our healing paths. I release all fears from any lifetime that could in any way block these light-filled, loving energies.*

Reading about these beings may help you to identify them when and if they show up. However, if you feel an affinity towards one or another, call in those beings' energy to begin to learn how it looks and feels. Ask these beings to show or tell you how they work and what they specifically do. Ask when you might call on them. In these ways you develop your own relationship with these beings. You may even invite them into your presence right now as you read about them.

Although I have worked with various Lightbeings for almost twenty years, it is difficult to describe them in words. I have developed an intimacy with each that goes far beyond the capacity of language. Instead, I know them through feelings and senses of their vibrations, powers and colors. I will do my best here to explain who they are and how they work. The following information is based both on what I have been taught, as well as what I have experienced. Please note that the entire process is subjective and given to each of us from our own individual personality and unique perspective.

SPIRIT GUIDES

Every person and animal on the planet has one or more spirit guides. These beings travel with the individual over many, if not all, lifetimes. When I was much younger, a psychic friend of mine told me that in other incarnations I have been the spirit guide for the being who is currently my spirit guide. We take turns guiding each other.

Spirit guides hold space as teachers, advisors, and supporters, understanding each person's soul work: his mission, challenges, obstacles, and path to ascension. Most of the work of the guides and the Divine Self is communicated in the dream state, and manifests while awake.

During a healing session, the guides hold the big picture and call in the healing team, which may include the elohim, ascended masters, archangels, angels and alien Lightbeings.

Foundations of Energy Healing

THE RAYS OF LIGHT

Much has been written about the Rays of Light, and I include them here now to explain the connection between the ascended masters and archangels and their powers and qualities. The Rays of Light are vectors of intention and manifestations of intellectual, creative and social expressions. Each ray is the embodiment/ expression of one of the great God-Qualities, such as Divine Will, Divine Wisdom, Divine Love, and so on, designed to enlighten the planet.

A *chohan* (or lord) of a ray is an ascended master who has been placed in charge of one of the rays, due to having an extraordinary natural spiritual affinity for that ray. Each spiritual being anchors the energies of the rays on different planes, and each plane is related to the frequency of change and societal growth. Each one is integral to the experiences of humanity living on the planet. They influence reality and society in order to make up the playing field that we call life. It is said that we, as individuals, come in to all of our incarnations on the same ray. On the next page is a chart that shows the links between the rays, the ascended masters and the archangels.

ELOHIM

The elohim (translated from Hebrew, meaning "All That God Is") are the highest level of angelic beings. They work on major global issues, and have come to us in this time to assist us with the expansion of our energy bodies during this transformation. Biblically, the elohim are the creator gods, the beings God created to help Him create the universe. In some teachings, the elohim are described as the thought attributes of God, whereas the angels are called the feelings of God.

I have witnessed the presence of the elohim in a session even when I think an issue is fairly mundane. Their presence lets me

46

The Spiritual Healing Team

RAY	COLOR	CHOHAN	ARCHANGEL	QUALTITIES
First	Blue	El Morya	Michael	Protection, power, initiative
Second	Yellow	Kuthumi	Jophiel	Illumination, wisdom, perception
Third	Pink	Paul the Venetian	Chamuel	Love, tolerance, gratitude
Fourth	White	Sarapis Bay	Gabriel	Purity, resurrection, artistic development
Fifth	Green	Hilarion	Raphael	Concentration, truth, scientific discovery
Sixth	Red	Jesus	Uriel	Devotional worship, ministration, peace
Seventh	Violet	St. Germain	Zadkiel	Ordered service, culture, refinement, diplomacy, invocation

know that what seems mundane from an emotional level is really connected to a much more universal shift. For instance,

I recently conducted a distance healing for a group with the express intention to clear the mental body from worry and anxiety. Rapture Elohim entered the session and began to unzip tension from the heart of the participants. She placed a different crystal on each person in the group to address his or her own particular emotional issues. Rapture's presence in the session, with her particular job being to "redeem all parts of our wholeness so it can communicate and co-create," conveyed to me that these participants' mental constructs of worry and anxiety go far beyond the individual. In fact these feelings are endemic—an indication of a much larger vibration of global worry attached to these times of intense change.

Foundations of Energy Healing

JJ Wilson at Alchemical Mage, who provided me with express permission to share the following, describes the elohim in the following ways:

- **Alpha Omega Elohim** looks like an opalescent sphere of Light. She divides into two spheres and a vesica pisces is created where they intersect. This vesica pisces is the Alpha Omega Threshold, a Beginning and an Ending. This creates the arena required for a universe, a dimension, a game such as this one, or a lifetime.

- **Faith Elohim** looks like a vertical column of white Light shot through with gold. The energy moves in both directions. She focuses the connection with God that Hope has opened. Faith is the requirement for action and expression of this inner relationship to Divinity.

- **Grace Elohim** looks like iridescent snow falling in spirals. She creates a complete break from the past and a fresh start in each Now moment. Like a Divine lubricant, her energy unlocks blockages in all of the bodies and ends all past referencing.

- **Harmony Elohim** looks like opalescent planes of all the Rays sparkling within white Light. Harmony creates connections between all octaves of Creation through music and color spectrums. She can reveal the next octave of any experience, feeling, thought, skill, perception, vision or probability and requires the opening of consciousness for harmonization with that next octave.

- **Hope Elohim** looks like very pale blue Light shot through with gold that manifests as an inward moving spiral formation. She sanctifies your relationship to Divinity. Her frequency allows you to feel close to God even when you are lonely or sad.

The Spiritual Healing Team

- *Liberty Elohim* looks like a shimmering, scintillating wall of iridescent indigo, violet, silver, copper, and turquoise Light. Liberty purifies and dismantles obsolete reality constructs and assists you to cross the Thresholds of Creator and Creation with ecstasy.

- *Love Elohim* looks like soft pink Light shot through with gold that manifests as an outward moving spiral formation. Hope, Faith and Love synergistically work together. Love takes Hope's childlike connection to God and the unshakable focus of Faith and radiates it outward to All Life. She redeems the Oneness of Creation through a constant outpouring of the experience of communion with Source.

- *Mercy Elohim* looks like waves of flowing, highly iridescent greens of every imaginable and unimaginable hue. As Harmony opens consciousness into the next octaves of perception, we often judge parts of our wholeness as unworthy. Mercy purifies the judgment and the feelings of unworthiness and lifts us so that we can consciously and fully open to our true place in the universe.

- *Peace Elohim's* energy is a radiant pearlescent white. As Harmony reveals and requires the next octaves, and Mercy purifies and lifts us to our proper positioning to those octaves, Peace completely fills and opens us at all levels. She opens all of the Gateways of the Divine Names, within and without, so that we may be redeemed throughout the Many Mansion Worlds of Light.

- *Purity Elohim* looks like bands of parallelograms made of blue-ultraviolet light. Darkness and trauma are just condensed Light. Purity expands the condensation and then, very gently, dissolves old traumas and orientations from the bodies, purifying all of the parts of your wholeness so that they can vibrate at the same frequency.

- *Rapture Elohim* looks like iridescent metallic honey, all the Rays blended together just before they go to white Light. Grace, Purity and Rapture work closely together. Once structures are unlocked, obsolete structures are dissolved, and everything is fully in the Now, Rapture redeems all parts of your wholeness so it can communicate and co-create.

- **Victory Elohim** looks like gold-white Light radiating in all directions. Throughout all of Creation, Victory Elohim recalls all of the layers of individuation and separation back into Oneness, so that individuals may understand their personal ascension process as it is connected to a much vaster program of universal ascension.

ARCHANGELS

Archangels serve larger areas of human life, and so are sometimes called overlighting angels. They often come into healing sessions and make powerful, overarching changes that may clear issues throughout many of the client's lifetimes.

Each archangel is associated with a Ray of Light and a power. The chart on page 47 lists the seven primary archangels, with their commonly taught colors and powers. However, I have also felt and worked with a few others, including archangels Ariel and Metatron, and I have heard of others such as Remiel, Haniel, Ratziel, and Saraqael as well.

Some healers specifically call on the archangels for their support. For instance, Raphael may be called upon to heal issues on the mental/emotional levels, and Michael is used for powerful clearings and cutting chords. I have called on specific archangels, and I have witnessed them coming into sessions on their own as needed. The way I understand this is that I do not consider that I know all the aspects that are unfolding in each healing so I am not in charge of calling in each Lightbeing who can help. Most of the work is being done on the spiritual plane beyond my comprehension and therefore beings show up as needed per the clients' guides.

The Spiritual Healing Team

ASCENDED MASTERS

*I am a brother of yours, who has travelled a little
longer upon the Path than has the average student, and
has therefore incurred greater responsibilities. I am
one who has wrestled and found his way into a greater
measure of light than has the aspirant who will read
this article, and I must therefore act as a transmitter of
the light, no matter what the cost... My work is to teach
and spread the knowledge of the Ageless Wisdom
wherever I can find a response, and I have been doing
this for many years.*[2]

So says the Tibetan, the ascended master who channels the
teachings of Alice Bailey's book *A Treatise on White Magic or The
Way of the Disciple* (1934). Alice Bailey described the majority of
her work, written between 1919 and 1949, as having been
telepathically dictated to her by a Master of Wisdom, initially
referred to only as "the Tibetan" or by the initials "D.K.," later
identified as Ascended Master Djwal Khul. Her writings were of
the same nature as those of Madame Blavatsky and came to be
known as the "Ageless Wisdom Teachings."

We get most of our contemporary information about the
ascended masters from these two women. Ascended masters are
believed to be spiritually enlightened beings who in past incarnations were ordinary humans, but who have undergone a series of
spiritual transformations.

Ascended masters are often incarnated and even exist today.
They are old souls, having lived so many times that they have
become self-realized. That is, they have successfully united their
hearts, minds and divine wills, and they are now teachers.

When the ascended masters enter my sessions, it is often to
provide information and wisdom to the client, as well as to
recommend spiritual practices that relate to mastery. As with the
archangels, I call them in when I am privy to exactly what issue
my client is dealing with. As an example, Saint Germain works
with the Violet Flame, an energetic process that clears all
negativity, old issues and energetic sludge from our fields. I ask
for the Violet Flame when a client's fields feel heavy or dense.

Foundations of Energy Healing

ANGELS

Angels work with humans on all aspects of Life. The ones that I have dealt with the most in my healing practice are the angels of healing, protection, transformation, prosperity, and emotional distress. Some sources say that angels can incarnate as humans, and, on occasion, it is possible for humans to enter into the angelic kingdom. However, for the most part, it is said that angels have never been human beings.

As such, angels work on all levels of creation. They are the worker bees under the direction of the archangels. Each person has a guardian angel who watches over and protects. They do all the work: clear energy, pull out trauma, repair the energy bodies and grid, bring in lightcodes, remove entities, soothe our hearts and minds, help us ground and more. The list of possibilities is as unlimited as the number of angels in the other dimensions!

As always, use your subtle senses to discern who arrives. Angels often come in groups. Although they don't literally have wings, you may see or feel a sense of wings or expansive light. Alternately, I have seen tiny angelic beings who easily move in and out of small areas of the body. You may choose to ask for an angel to come to you so you can begin to notice how they look or feel. They long to communicate, so ask a lot of questions to develop your own relationship with each.

ALIEN LIGHTBEINGS

Yes, aliens do exist, although I have been told that they prefer to be called Lightbeings. Some alien Lightbeings include the Plaeidians, Hathors, Lyrans, Siriuns, Ashtar Command, the Federation of Light, and the Federation of Councils. Honestly, I have never met a Lightbeing who has not been of the Light and filled me with Love.

The Spiritual Healing Team

I have seen them look like tall, regal men in robes, hooded entities, thin, waif-like feminine beings, and those with beetle-like bodies and dog-like faces. I have seen a group of Lightbeings who look like six male figures in robes each trailing a different color of light behind them enter my sessions and meditations many times. Plus there are many accounts of an alien race that looks like our lizards.

The ones who join us in our healing sessions are higher-level beings assigned to assist us with our ascension. I have seen them doing "psychic surgery" on clients, literally transforming and transmuting physical organs, ailments, and symptoms. Many offer information for further growth to the client. Others bring in "new" technologies and ideas that we have not worked with before.

One of my clients was a 45-year-old man who suffered a brain injury during a fall fifteen years ago. Although he was able to function fairly normally, he had a hard time making decisions and thinking linearly. He also seemed to procrastinate more than was reasonable and I was not sure if this was another symptom of the injury.

During one session, a number of Lightbeings entered the session. I saw and felt them working deep in his lumbar spine, rewiring the communication system there. Upon completion of that task, they moved into his brain, and rewired nerves and message centers in his brain. His wife was in the room as well, and I have to admit that I thought she was going to think I was crazy if I told her this, but I said it anyway.

The next day I received word from the both of them letting me know that on the night of the session the husband had to write a letter to a business client of his. He managed to do so in half the time it normally took him, and with more grace and ease than they had witnessed since before his accident. They were amazed and thrilled.

Personally, I love it when alien beings enter my sessions because I always know that they will be using techniques and technology that I do not have access to on this planet. However, if you ever have any concern about whether beings are of the Light, simply ask them if they are. Be clear that you work only with those beings of the Light. If they are not benevolent, they will leave.

HOME PRACTICE

As you practice running sessions with clients, friends and your pets, take note:

- How do you know what to do next?

- Did an inspiration or idea pop into your mind? Or did you merely flow from one thing to the next?

- If it was an inspiration or idea, was it a thought or a message? How do you tell them apart?

- Do you feel or see the presence of others?

As you practice being more aware of your process, you will gain clarity and confidence.

ENDNOTES: CHAPTER 4

1. Joshua David Stone, Ph.D., The Ascended Masters Light the Way: Beacons of Ascension (Flagstaff: Light Technology Publishing, 1995), p. 206.

2. Alice A. Bailey, *A Treatise on White Magic*, (New York: Lucis Publishing company, 1934), "Extract form a Statement by the Tibetan," p. vii.

5. Anatomy of a Healing Session

What if healing was based upon trust, rapport
and love instead of education, credentials,
specialization and licensure?

As we begin to work with subtle energy, it is helpful to develop tools to assist us in our work. Energy healing relies on building a trust of our extrasensory perception, and our skills mature over time. This chapter outlines the tools that have helped me train my senses. Included in this chapter are:

- Aligning energetically with your clients

- Setting intentions

- Using muscle testing to check your intuition

- Asking the spiritual healing team questions to get your instructions

- Creating healthy boundaries, and

- Protecting your energy field and your space

ESTABLISH ALIGNMENT

In my practice, I usually sit (or speak on the phone) with my clients before we begin a healing session so I can ask what their intentions are for the session. During this time, I quiet my mind and open myself up to receiving energetic information. I psychically look at the energy body to see if I am drawn to any inconsistencies in the physical body. I use my intuition to look for patterns in the client's personal relationships in this and past lifetimes, which I *see* as highlighted images in my mind's eye. I look for karmic ties, which come to me as a *knowing* that this is related to a past life. I do all this to clue in to what this session will focus on.

These are my first impressions. For me this is a subtle experience, born from many years of practice. The healing actually begins during this time, as the energetic connection between the client and myself is established. I have already begun to move into an altered state of consciousness. I release all thoughts and rely on guidance from my sixth sense. This puts us both into a more relaxed state, even if it's an almost imperceptible change. The resonance between us has begun.

The true underlying causes of whatever the client is concentrating on will become apparent as the session continues. There are always issues and memories that will be hidden from his mind, or that he is avoiding. Listening closely to the spiritual healing team, I am always guided about what to bring to the client's attention and what to keep to myself.

I continue this ritual once we formally begin the healing process. Following is a recommendation, based on much trial and error over the years, of how to align with your client and your team at the beginning of a session.

- **Take a moment to breathe and ground yourself into your body.** Being anchored firmly in your body is the best and most accurate way to channel the spiritual healing team's Light. The more grounded and centered you are, the more you are a strong conduit of the energies.

- **Expand your energy field by setting the intention to do so.** I like to use the internal command: "I expand my field to the size of this state. I expand my field to the size of this country. I expand my field to the size of this planet." This, for me, feels like a slight relaxation of the space around me. Once you feel it open up, set the intention that Earth energy

moves up and through your field, grounding and flushing it.
This allows the beings of the Universe to assist you in the
session. I visualize my feet firmly planted in the Earth, with
lush tropical vines growing up and around my feet and legs,
tenderly drawing me down while simultaneously energizing
me. I allow these vines to continue up the rest of my body,
gently wrapping around me and holding me in a loving
embrace. After some practice, this preparation becomes
natural and almost instantaneous.

■ **Connect to your client.** Perhaps put your hands on her
shoulders. Move your awareness into her body. Notice what
stands out to you. Notice to where your attention is drawn.
You may begin to feel things in your own body, like aches
and pains, pressure, or emotions. By the way, this works the
same way whether your client is a person, an animal, a plant
or the Earth.

This works similarly when you and your client are at a
distance. With a quiet mind, connect to your client, either
visually or viscerally, by stating, "I now connect to _____
(client's name)." It may help to look at a picture of that
person and/or to know his birthday, address, or anything that
helps you focus on him. Then notice which part of his body
or energy field you are drawn to. Notice if you feel sensations
in your own body. Maintain the connection by consciously
returning your awareness to this image, body, and all the
sensations.

You may not feel anything in your own body. Whatever
works for you is fine. Don't do anything with this
information yet. Just receive impressions. Never diagnose or
judge what your see and feel. And remember that you are just
getting information here. Energy is not contagious, it is
merely informative.

■ **Connect to your spiritual healing team.** Either tell them
that you are connecting, or simply set the intention to
connect. Wait until you see or feel the connection.
I make my mental connection with my team by rolling my

eyes up. The act of rolling the eyes up moves us into an altered state of consciousness, slowing the brainwaves from beta (conscious alert), to alpha (meditative) and theta (deeper meditative). Theta waves are strong during times of internal focus, meditation, prayer, and spiritual awareness. According to Connee Chandler, "Looking up encourages the brain to produce the kind of waves accessed in higher states of consciousness. Also, looking up tends to stimulate the pineal gland."[1]

I have found, over the years, that it is easier for me to see, feel and hear the Lightbeings when I shift my consciousness in this way.

I also invite my client's Higher Self and guides into the process. I can usually discern visually who has come in. Once the entire team has collected, I let go of trying to know who is doing what and ask for guidance from the group as a whole. Notice, if possible, who has arrived. Feel free to ask who is there. If need be, muscle test (explained below) to see if who you think is there really is there.

As always, this works well for me, but it may not work well for you. Use what feels natural and leave the rest. The only important message here is to create a consistent system of connection and communication that establishes you as a strong and reliable conduit of the etheric energies that are available to you.

HOME PRACTICE

Practice the following heart-to-heart connection with a friend or partner.

Sit on the floor cross-legged or in chairs with your feet on the floor. Sit close enough so that your knees are touching. Close your eye and breathe for 2 minutes. Quiet your mind.

Open your eyes and look directly into your friend's eyes. Place your right hands on each other's hearts. Stay in that position for up to five minutes.

- Focus on feeling into your friend's heart.
- Focus on seeing what is happening in hers or her energy field.
- Focus on picking up on one new thing about your friend... one thing you did not know before.

After the five minutes are up, share with each other what you felt and saw. Do not be surprised to notice how much you were able to pick up on and how accurate you were.

SET INTENTIONS

In essence, the goal of this kind of healing work is to move energy. Energy follows thought, or intention, so setting the intentions for the healing is of primary importance. Without this clarity, there is no direct path for the energy to move and flow.

Begin by taking the time to talk to your client about why he has come. What are the issues at hand? What would he like to uncover? What would he like to heal? The more detailed you can help your client be, the better, because it assures that you, the client and the healing team are in perfect alignment. So rather than setting a vague intention such as "Let's help my client feel better," be more specific with something like, "Let's heal the root cause of his migraine headache."

As you listen, it is easy to assume you understand what is being said. However, it has been my experience that people can often use words they think mean one thing, while I think they mean something else. For example, I once had a new client schedule a past life regression. I have done past life regressions for many years, and I have a specific process for that. When he came in, however, he really wanted to learn what his career path should be. In an effort to please him, I decided that I would regress him to a previous lifetime so he could see what his career was then. My mistake was that I did not communicate properly to him that the intention he set when he made the appointment and what he was asking for in the present were two different things. Needless to say, the session was frustrating for both of us, and he did not get his needs met.

I now take my time explaining the differences between contacting the guides for information and advice and uncovering information from the past. I also explain that it is not possible to accurately foretell the future. There is an infinite number of potential futures based on the infinite number of decisions we may make. Each decision sets its own course. So while you may see one possibility, it is based on the situation as it is in the present moment. The guides, however, see the broader view, so may have suggestions to help the client achieve momentum along her soul path.

Communication is key. Help your clients set clearly defined objectives by repeating back to them what they say, not what you think they are saying. Ask enough questions until you are clear that you are both speaking the same language. When this occurs, it is as if the intention becomes a laser beam. The result is that the soul is in alignment with the mind and the guides understand clearly, so that the most perfect spiritual healing team is gathered together and miracles occur!

MUSCLE TESTING

Communicating with your guides and the healing team is not always foolproof. Even after you have developed strong connections with them, there are times when answers will be unclear, the information murky. During those times, it can be most helpful to use a system that will help you determine the accuracy of answers to Yes/No questions.

Muscle testing—or kinesiology—is simple, straightforward and utilized by practitioners for a variety of analyses. Everyone can do it, because it is a process that helps us connect to our innate intelligence by using the body's electrical system and muscles. Besides discerning "Yes" and "No," it can be used to test for all health-related issues, such as the use of supplements, medications, tinctures, and treatments, as well as uncovering food allergies or sensitivities, and more.

The way it works is this: the human body, and everything else on the planet, have an electrical frequency. Any time a negative influence (whether that influence is physical, mental, emotional, or from some other source) is introduced to a body (either physically on the body or anywhere in the body's energy field), the electrical system will immediately be affected and the muscles will weaken. So when pressure is applied to a muscle, it cannot hold its strength. Our energy fields are so sensitive and so attuned to our surroundings that this recognition takes place within a nanosecond. Conversely, when something that is supportive or in any way helpful to the body is held anywhere in the body's energy field, the muscles will strengthen and hold strong.

Muscle testing has been around for centuries. It was brought into modern holistic practices in 1964, when chiropractor George Goodheart began to teach a kind of muscle testing that he called "Applied Kinesiology." His method of diagnosis and treatment was based on the belief that various muscles are linked to particular organs and glands, and that specific muscle weakness can signal distant internal problems such as nerve damage, reduced blood supply, chemical imbalances or other organ or gland dysfunction. Since then, applied kinesiology has been used as a diagnostic tool in numerous ways.

Here is a typical example of muscle testing in a chiropractor's office: you are given an herb or other supplement to hold in your non-dominant hand. You extend the other arm at a 90-degree angle from your body and are asked to keep it straight. The practitioner presses down on this arm and the opposite shoulder with equal pressure. If the herb is something you need, you will be able to resist the downward pressure and hold your arm rigid. If not, your dominant arm will weaken and the chiropractor will be able to push it down. The same procedure can be used to determine how often you should take each herb and the dosage each time.

Using an extended arm becomes impractical during many energy sessions. That's why, when using muscle testing in my practice, I have found the easiest way is to use my own hands.

The technique works by pressing your thumb and pinky on the non-dominant hand together. This creates a temporary closed circuit of your electrical system. There are two major electrical systems going through the arm: the first runs down the inside of the arm through the thumb and first three fingers, and the second goes down the outside of the arm and into the pinky. Pressing them together creates a strong electrical connection. There are three options here: pressing the tips of the thumb and pinky together, resting the thumb on top of the nail of the pinky, or pressing the pads of the fingers together.

The index finger of the dominant hand is used to gently try to pull the thumb and pinky apart to test whether this is a positive or negative response—in essence, testing the strength of the electrical current.

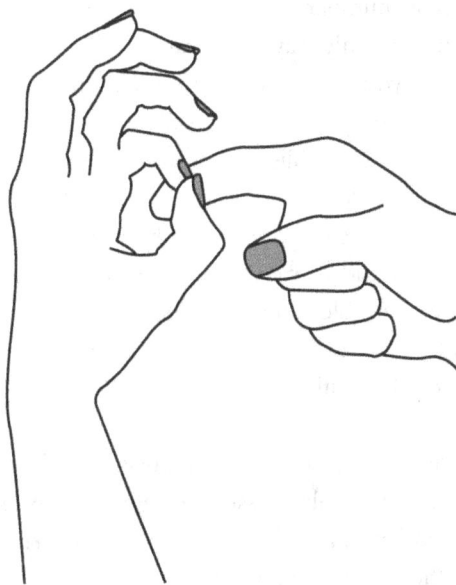

Muscle testing by pressing tips of thumb and pinky together.

I use muscle testing during my sessions initially to make sure I am connected to my team and, at times, to discern what's required of me, as well as to verify messages. I also use this to ask about essences, supplements, or types of treatment for my clients by acting as a proxy for them. (You may be more drawn to use a pendulum or any other way of receiving confirmation. This works the same way, so use the technique with which you are most comfortable.)

First and foremost, I clear my mind of all thought, as well as all attachment to the answers. The reason for this is that the muscle test picks up imperceptible nuances in the energy system of the body. Remember, our body's electrical system registers electrical current, created by thoughts, intentions and expectations, in a nanosecond. So wishing for or hoping for or even assuming about a "Yes" response will undoubtedly garner a "Yes" response. The number one rule then is: clear your mind of all expectation. The only way to guarantee valid information is to be able to make yourself an empty vessel, and not "impose" your own beliefs or energy into the process.

Once clear, I establish a strong connection to the client's body or energy field. I do this by focusing all of my attention on that person—her energy field or physical body. I set the clear intention to psychically move myself into the client's energy field. This is a perceptible, albeit subtle, change. I literally feel my energy shift a bit and then I know I am connected. (I often double-check that with a muscle test: *Am I connected to Brian? Yes or No?*)

I muscle test on my own hand, using the index finger of my dominant hand to apply pressure to the connection made with my thumb and index finger on my non-dominant hand (inside of the circle). If the connection holds strong, that is a "Yes." If the connection breaks, that is a "No."

When I am in a session and I receive guidance in the form of a signal or message, I often test its validity using this process. I want to be as clear as I can be that my thinking mind isn't coming up with ideas, but that, indeed, these are guided messages.

If you don't feel comfortable using muscle testing during a session, there are many other options for this kind of Yes/No communication. For instance, ask your team to show you the words "Yes" and "No" in your mind's eye. Or ask them to send the feelings for "Yes" and "No" into your body. And, again, make sure that you are taking yourself and your ego out of the process.

If you choose to use a pendulum instead, one can be made with any slightly heavy object at the end of a string or chain, although most people prefer using a crystal hanging from a chain. Before relying on it, ask your team to show you which direction it will move in when the answer is a "Yes," and which direction it will move in when the answer is a "No."

Choose whichever method is most comfortable for you. The only important thing here is to develop a simple and effective method of communication between yourself and your guides and healing team. Please remember to set your ego—and brilliant, creative, thinking mind—aside when seeking and receiving answers.

HOME PRACTICE

Design a series of Yes/No questions to practice muscle testing on yourself.

Practice quieting your mind and detaching yourself from what you think the answer is and allow your body and Higher Self to be the guides.

- My name is (use correct name).
- My name is (use incorrect name).
- I love ice cream.
- I need vitamins.
- I need more exercise.
- I am allergic to ....

Find the way that best suits you: using your finger, a pendulum, the sensations in your body, or picturing the words "Yes" and "No."

ASK QUESTIONS

During one healing session, my client and I were joined by one of the ascended masters. At the time, I wasn't able to discern who it was, but I saw the letter M. I told my client to look up Ascended Master M. He later reported to me that he did a search for M and found nothing related to the Ascended Masters. I then spent some time in quiet meditation and asked who it was who joined us, and received the information that it was Master Chohan. When I told this to my client, he asked how I knew. He was surprised to hear that I had just asked, as he never would have thought to do that.

Learning to communicate with the spirit world is like learning a new language. At the beginning, you may receive a single picture or a word from out of nowhere. Be patient as your conscious mind learns to translate their language. Stay strong in your desire to communicate, stay open to however the communication comes, and the guides will continue with their best efforts.

If you see a picture, image or color and you do not understand it, ask for clarity. If a feeling moves through you and it is confusing as to whose it is or what to do with it ask for clarity.

When I was first practicing receiving messages and answers in my mediations, the incoming information was vague. I would say, "Show me in pictures, please. Pictures are easiest for me." Slowly my guides and I began developing the language in pictures and images that my sensory system could best translate. From there, my other senses of hearing, smell, and knowing developed.

When I began channeling the Federation of Councils, it took time as my Higher Self worked with them to develop an accurate language system. For months, they worked on attuning a psychic channel, or tunnel, that traveled from my brow and ear chakras to them. There were many times during this process that, when I asked the Federation of Councils a question, before they responded, I could feel, see and sense a group of them conferring as to how best to answer. It taught me that they had to figure out how to translate their comprehension of the question at hand into a language I could understand. Once the channel was fully attuned, however, the incoming information flowed effortlessly and I was able to verbalize their ideas without thought or question.

Intuition

Intuition is the innate connection between us and other worlds. As we move into the higher dimensions, the acknowledgment and awareness of these other worlds expands. Intuition is the open door to communicating.

Intuition is governed by the right side of the brain, the side that holds our memories, feelings, dreams and imagination. When the very first bit of information comes in—via a vision, feeling or knowing—and you interpret it in a nanosecond without analysis, it flows easily. But it is easy to stop the flow of information by questioning it. When you say, "No, that can't be true," it's gone. When you say, "I don't know what is happening," it's gone. When you tell yourself you can't do this, the information does not come through.

Everybody receives intuitive information differently. The four core types of intuition are *clairvoyance* (seeing images or pictures), *clairaudience* (hearing the words), *clairsentience* (feeling) and *claircognizance* (knowing it all at once). However, any of the five senses may be used—a number of people receive smells or tastes, too.

Clairvoyants see into other dimensions. There are different types of this kind of vision. Some people report seeing through physical objects, such as walls and envelopes. Some people see illness and disease in others' energy fields. Some see future events and possibilities, while others see into the past. The way the information is perceived is also varied. Some clairvoyants see other people or spirits as if they were physically present, while others see them in their mind's eye.

Clairaudients hear sounds, music and voices not of the physical world. Hearing the sounds of angels, disembodied voices and warnings are common for clairaudients. Some of these sounds and voices seem internal and others external. As clairaudients become more adept with their gift, the sounds come on command, as direct answers to questions, rather than as randomly occurring events.

Clairsentience is the experience of nonphysical sense perception. Empaths are clairsentient, picking up on the feelings of others. It is also common to feel information, interpreting it through a fleeting impression, a brief image or a gut reaction. When people first recognize their clairsentient gifts, it may be difficult to discern if sensations or emotions are theirs or someone else's. With practice, that clarity is established.

Claircognizance is less common, and is the ability to see the big picture. Those with this gift are able to see or understand how an issue came to be and what the connections are from the past and present, and possibly even in the future. It is considered to be a *mental* psychic ability, which focuses on holistic (whole) understanding.

We each receive our intuitive messages from a combination of any of these, and it may even change over time. It is fun to begin to discern how you are picking up information. Do you see your guides, feel them, hear their words? Or is it a combination of all of that? Once you are clear how the information comes to you, you can then communicate more efficiently with your guides by asking them to "speak" to you in the most effective ways.

For me, my thoughts are centered on one side or the other, and guidance enters down the middle of the back of my head. When I work with the Federation, I roll my eyes up and slightly to the right. That is how they enter. When I am in a healing session, I often imagine that my crown chakra has lines of light that go straight up, and I set my intention to open my crown for incoming information.

Remember that many of our guides have not had lives on this planet, or if they did, they may not remember how inconsistent it can be when we first start using our extrasensory perceptions. As you develop your relationship with your guides and healing team, asking for what you need is key. Respectfully let them know how best to communicate (in pictures, words or ideas), what your boundaries are around your healing work (for instance, what kind of clients you want and don't want), how many people you want to see a week, and so on.

The Spiritual Healing Team has been clear with me that they are honored to assist us as we work to help our fellow human beings and the planet. To say they love helping us is an understatement, because they are All Loving and All Knowing and want nothing more than to help us ascend into the greatest expression of ourselves! Therefore, ask for their help and guidance all along the way.

During a Session

Any time the information exchange between you and your healing team is unclear, don't worry and don't get frustrated. Start asking questions or giving your healing team prompts. I often ask questions like: "Do you want me to sit here, or would you like me to move?" "Shall I move this energy or keep my hands still?" "Are you finished with this?" Or I prompt: "Show me where you want me."

There are all sorts of reasons a communication breakdown may occur:

- **The client's energy field is hazy.**
  There's not much you can do about this except to trust your intuition. Know, too, that you are never alone, and the guides and healing team have shown up. Relax your mind and allow your hands to move where they will.

- **You got distracted.**
  This happens, no worries. Take a breath, re-ground and direct your attention back to your client's body and the healing team. Ask to be shown (or told) what they are doing, and ask for guidance.

HOME PRACTICE

Since everyone receives information differently, and
even that changes over time, practice asking
questions of your guides and trying these techniques. It is likely that one suits you more readily
than another:

Automatic writing
Begin by sitting quietly, holding a pen and paper.
Center your mind and body. Ask your guides a
question and put the pen to the paper. Allow your
hand to write without holding back, without
judgment. Read what you've written after it is
complete.

"Mind-Mapping"
This is somewhat similar to automatic writing but
instead of using a pen and paper, use colored
markers and a large pad. Allow your hand to write,
draw and connect images. Use the colors that you
are drawn to. Use the entire paper. This technique
allows the creativity of your right brain to take
over, reducing the rational thinking of the left brain.
Allow information and messages to flow, without
censorship. Interpret the finished product.

Looking for signs
Signs from the subconscious can be manifest in
common places. I know of people who see their
signs on license plates, hear them in the lyrics of
songs on the radio, find them while turning to
random pages in books, or receive them from a
random passerby.

Write down your dreams
A great number of people have prophetic or
intuitive dreams. Keep a record of your dreams so
you can decipher what your subconscious mind and
Higher Self are telling you.

Anatomy of a Healing Session

- **The work is being done at a very high level, in the outer dimensions.**
  Sometimes when work is being done in the outer limits of the client's energy field (think 8 feet or more out), I lose sight of it. I then kick my other senses into gear, feeling, hearing or knowing what is taking place. Alternatively, when that fails, I relax and trust the process, and wait for further instructions.

- **Your energy field fluctuated.**
  This can occur when you get worried, when you're triggered by something you feel or see during the session, or when you question yourself. The fluctuation may result in a headache, a pulsing of the third eye, feeling groggy or getting hot. If any of these occur, widen your energy field again, and call on the Earth energy to rise into your field, bringing with it all the support available to you.

  Take notice when this happens so you can explore it later, on your own. Sometimes your energy field fluctuation will be the result of a triggering that is more about you than the client. This can be a tremendous gift (from your client and the healing team) for you. But resolve to just quickly notice it in that moment, and wait until you are doing your own work to "unwrap" that gift.

- **You are thinking, or making this a mental process.**
  Similar to why your energy field would fluctuate, the same goes for any time you make this a mental, left-brain process. This work is not a left-brain method, so trying to "figure it out" pulls you away from the senses available to you from your right brain.

CREATE HEALTHY BOUNDARIES

We are in control of our energy input and output. Practicing setting healthy energetic boundaries, activating and aligning our chakras, cleansing our fields after sessions and clearing the workspace are important tools to add to our healing skills.

Foundations of Energy Healing

The human energy field exists about 14 feet in diameter around us. So if you are in a normal-sized room with someone else, your energy fields are intersecting. In fact, we intersect with others' energy fields all the time: walking by people in a store; driving past them on the road; sitting next to them on public transportation, and so on. Because of this close contact, it is normal to pick up on other people's feelings and thoughtforms.

A thoughtform is created when we repeat a particular thought over and over again. The thought, which initiates as pure energy, solidifies into an "energetic cloud" that is, quite simply, beginning to manifest into matter. The thoughtform becomes a belief that we hold onto, which colors our perceptions of reality.

Sensing others' feelings and thoughtforms is called *empathy*. It is very common, especially when setting the intention to connect with someone else, that you will empathize with whatever is in his or her energy field. That can become problematic, however, when their negative beliefs resonate with negative beliefs of your own.

For instance, if a client is sad about a relationship that just ended, and I feel that sadness after she leaves, many people would say that it is because her sadness is now in my field. Actually, it means that her sadness vibrated at the same frequency as a sadness that lives within me already. This is an opportunity for me to recognize the issues that may still need to be resolved and healed within myself. More often than not, we get clients who "trigger" us in this way all the time. Our souls always draw to us the people and situations that provide us with the greatest opportunities to heal our own fears, traumas or issues. More will be said about this in the next chapter.

Healthy boundaries empower us to stay aware of sudden, unsettling feelings. Create your boundaries by setting conscious intentions. First, affirm your intentions to your guides and the Universe by stating: "I am the power and cause of all of my feelings, attitudes and emotions. I am completely protected from other people's negative (or heavier or denser or darker) energies."

Anatomy of a Healing Session

Second, stay consciously aware of sudden changes in your feelings and energy levels. Check in to where you feel the changes occurring in your body and notice which chakra is affected. Re-energize and realign that chakra by filling it with a beautiful bubble of light in that chakra's color. Then visualize the chakra (and if that is not possible for you to do, merely use your imagination and set your intentions): move the chakra into vertical alignment with the others if it is off-center, and spin it clockwise.

A very quick way to clear your field whenever you have limited time, such as between sessions, is to stand up and plant your feet firmly on the ground. Raise your hands over your head. State "Release!" as you drop your arms quickly down to your sides, as if expelling the unwanted energy out of your body and into the Earth. Repeat three times.

Furthermore, if someone's energy field is filled with negativity, illness or "gunk" from their own lives or other people's lives, we can also feel it in ours. The result of that could be one or more of the following:

- Feeling suddenly sad, angry, fearful (or any similar kind of emotions)
- Feeling tired
- Having a stomachache or headache
- Becoming constipated
- Feeling energetically heavy or stuck
- Having strange dreams that don't feel like they connect to your life

If any of these issues persist, it is indicative of a similar issue that is held in your own emotional body. Following is a quick way to connect to your body-mind to identify and release the stuck issue.

Begin by quieting your mind and settling into your body. Using your muscle testing, ask:

"Did this issue occur when I was between the ages of one and five? Five and ten? Ten and fifteen?" etc. When your muscles test weakly that means you've hit the age-range of the trauma. Specify the age then by asking, "Eleven? Twelve? Thirteen?" etc.

Once you have the age, go back in your memory about everything you can remember about that year. Where did you live? Who lived in your home with you? What major events occurred that year? What minor events do you remember? Who was your teacher? Who were your friends? All of these can point to a situation that left an imprint on your psyche.

Don't be surprised if the issue you recall is similar to the issue you were working on healing in your client. Referring back to the relationship issue, you may realize that this was the year your parents divorced or you broke up with your first boyfriend, or had an issue with another kind of relationship, etc. This lets you know that you need to rethink your values and beliefs regarding, for instance, relationships, rejection, abandonment or holding your power. Alternately, it shows you that it is now time to release the hurt and forgive.

A WORD ABOUT PROTECTION

Protection is an interesting word, in that it brings with it a connotation of danger—something out there from which we must protect ourselves. In fact, energy is merely information. It is not dangerous or harmful. No one can "attack" or impair you in any way unless you agree to it on some level. When you are in contact with an uncomfortable energy—whether it is a thought-form, a negative entity, an illness—acknowledge it with curiosity and concern, remembering that you are in charge of your own energy field at all times.

Anatomy of a Healing Session

I have always been very clear with my guides that I am not interested in working with potentially violent or harmful people. I set that intention at the very beginning of my healing practice, knowing that I would be in a room alone with my clients. And my guides have always set that limit for me. I never get clients who are "sketchy" or who would potentially sue me, or anything like that. And because I know I am safe, I never turn people away.

Yet if you are ever in a situation where you feel vulnerable, claim your right to protect your field from unwanted input. One of the easiest ways to do this is to create a shield of Light. However you imagine your field to be is how it will be. Honestly, it's that simple. If you want a Teflon shield, you can have that... just make sure it is see-through. If you want a semi-permeable shield so you feel everything your client feels, you will get that. Decide what is best for you and create it.

I prefer a strong, see-through plastic shield that does not allow anything in and also sucks everything out. The way I create this is by saying to myself, "I now create a shield of Light around my field. This shield protects me from being affected by others' energies. This shield also acts as a vacuum, sucking out anything in my field that does not serve my highest good."

I picture it around me. And so it is.

Negative Entities

Yes, negative entities do exist. They are energies or lightbeings that vibrate at the low frequencies of negativity and thrive off of the negative energy we carry, such as fear, anger, guilt, and so on. They use these emotions as their "food," and so, through a co-creative agreement with us at the soul level, attach themselves to us and perpetuate these feelings so they can nourish themselves. They may be called negative astral energies, negative elementals, dark forces, demons, or parasites.

We all have these entities in our fields at one time or another. No one is a bad person for having them, and no one is to blame, because it is not a conscious connection. As Love is truly the only energy there is, and everything else is a different shade of that

HOME PRACTICE

Develop a daily practice of refreshing and clearing your energy field. One way to do this is in a meditation practice in which you connect to your heart.

Allow all the muscles around your heart to relax and soften as you breathe easily and deeply. Take the time to allow any pent up feelings to be expressed. Next, visualize an image of something that allows your heart to fill with love. This may be an experience you have had, or it may be another image, such as a kitten playing with a ball of yarn, a babbling brook, or a beautiful sunset. Whatever your image, see all the aspects of it and feel the emotions it evokes.

Now, notice how your body feels. It will tingle or vibrate slightly. Perhaps you may smile or even giggle. Will those feelings to spread into every cell of every muscle, bone, organ and gland of your body. Sit in those vibrations for ten minutes.

same color, so to speak, these beings are also originally from the Light and have somehow lost their way. Just as we suffer the farther we move away from the Light, so too are they (presumably) suffering.

It is best to remove these entities when found, and send them back to the Light. I have one teacher who said when she came across some kind of negative entity, she would merely flick it out of the client's energy field. I, however, prefer to ask Spirit to "release all energies, entities, thoughtforms, emotions, cellular memory, orientations, pictures of reality, devices, implants, intrusions and effects in my body and fields that are not of my core Divine essence." Use the ascended master Djwhal Khul or Archangel Michael to do this work, if you are so called. We have all the help we need from the higher realms. The entity release is included in Chapter 11, Energy Release Processes.

Cleansing Your Space

Over the years, I have learned a lot of tricks for cleansing my energy field and my space. I have adopted the ones that feel powerful and yet are simple for me, but of course, you may be drawn to other ones. Depending on whether you are drawn to Earth, air, fire or water energy, you will find the ways that suit your style. Native healing traditions have many tools and techniques of their own, while the more esoteric practices utilize others. All can work well, and, of course, it is the intention behind whatever you do that makes all the difference.

Here are a few ideas for keeping your energy field clean and aligned:

■ Take a bath in two cups of baking soda and one cup of Epsom salts (other salts may work just as well, like sea salt or other mineral bath salts, but try not to use those with artificial

HOME PRACTICE

Create a protective bubble around your energy field. Using your imagination, visualize or feel a bubble around your body. If it is easier for you, you can imagine your body inside of a bubble that is in front of you. Either way, give this bubble qualities:

- What is it made of?
- Is it see-through or opaque?
- Is it a color?
- How big is it?
- Do unwanted energies bounce off of it, or slide off of it?
- Can it vacuum out unwanted energies, too?

After you have made your bubble as specific as you can, notice how you feel inside of it. Notice how it feels to create a safe space for your energy field.

scents mixed in). You may choose to add essential oils or grape seed oil for your skin. Soak for 20 minutes.

- Juice with greens and fruit

- Tone

- Take a sauna or steam bath

- Drink water with lemon, three times a day

- Use flower essences, such as the Rose Trio for Healers, Caretaker, or The Healer's Toolbox, all found at Green Hope Farm (www.greenhopeessences.com)

Here are a few ideas for cleansing your office, home and healing space:

- Smudge with sage

- Draw Reiki symbols or sacred geometries in the air with incense

Anatomy of a Healing Session

- Drop Wild Sage essential oil on the massage table, desk or chair, or put some on a cotton ball or tissue and leave it in the room overnight. (Alternatively, use other essential oil blends specifically for clearing, such as Spells Out by AZ Alchemist Oils (alchemistoils.com) or Purification spray by Alaskan Flower Essences (alaskanessences.com)

- Tone

- Ring a crystal or Tibetan bowl

- In conjunction with your guides, create a grid of Light around the office/healing room that consistently cleanses the space

- Use the Home-Sweet-Home Enviro-Pack potions from Alchemical Mage. These potions are created through a process of channeling intense energy and sound (toning) into a pure, distilled water base

6. Facilitating an Energy Healing Session

What if we could actually be the conduits
of healing energy for another person?

Now that we have explored different ways to work with subtle energy, it is time to see how to facilitate a 4th-dimensional healing session. As the facilitator of this process, you hold the connection between the client and the healing team. You are acting as the conductor of the energies. According to physics, when pouring water into a glass, if there is a rod in the glass, like a straw or a spoon handle, the water will be attracted to the rod and will flow down it instead of spilling all over. When you set the intention to facilitate a healing session, you are that rod that attracts and funnels the higher vibrational energies.

The question may arise: *Am I doing the healing or is the healing energy merely coming through me?* The answer is "Yes" to both. Our role as the healer is to direct the energy, receive intuitive guidance and messages, support the client emotionally, and utilize whatever additional energy/bodywork/counseling training we have. At the same time, our higher selves work in conjunction with the spiritual healing team to manipulate energies in different dimensions.

I work with one healer who goes directly into trance and has no clear memories afterwards of what happened and why. She is adamant that all the healing energies come from her—her higher self and soul. She holds no belief that she is working with any kind of angels or spirits. I also know other healers who consider themselves to be conduits but not the actual healers. They remain passive throughout the session, merely holding space, while seeing and hearing what the spiritual healing team is doing.

When I work, I am a conscious channel, although in an altered state, able to discern images, various members of the healing team, changes in the Light, a person's energy grid, and more.

All ways work.

I have also spent many years not logically understanding a lot of what goes on in my healings. I could see it, but I didn't get it. I did what I was "told," but I didn't know why. And the healings worked anyway.

I used to do all my healings in silence, allowing my client to rest quietly during the session. From my years as a yoga instructor, I learned that a deep meditative state is the best condition for healing of any kind...anyone who has experienced Yoga Nidra may attest to that. At the end of the work, I always asked my clients if they would like to know what came up during the session. Invariably they would say "Yes," and I would relay back what I remembered.

However, I started narrating the sessions a few years ago, and had a lot of positive feedback from that. People like to feel involved with the process. I realized that talking about the issues allows clients to work through them consciously while the energy is shifted, cleared and healed. This adds a powerful layer to the process. It also adds trust, because when I tell them something they resonate with, they relax a bit more and trust me to take them where they need to go.

Some rules for speaking the session out loud include **never** speak in a judgmental voice about anything and **never** act shocked, surprised or scared. I have been to healers who do not adhere to this way of thinking, and I have left sessions afraid, in shock, or feeling judged or "wrong." As a healer, you have as much responsibility to hold safe space for your client as a therapist or doctor does. Therefore, please know that you may be witness to past abuse, crime, addiction, infidelity, as well as dark energies and entities. These are all part of the human condition and experience. At one point in time, in different lifetimes perhaps, we have all experienced these things, and we all learn from them. No experiences are better or worse than others. They are all just experiences. Please read more about this in Chapter 7, Clearing Trauma.

THE SESSION

Fourth-dimensional healing can be incorporated into any type of therapy or healing practice. Use this for your pets, your plants, and the planet, if you feel called to. The techniques are the same. And this work can effortlessly be done from a distance as well when we understand that time and space are a third-dimensional construct.

The healer's job is to continually move her awareness back and forth between her client's body, her own body and the healing team. As you practice, your skills and gifts will guide you to conduct your own sessions in the ways that are best suited to you. Be open to infinite possibilities!

If you are with your client, you may choose to begin a session by holding her head, or placing your hands on her shoulders. If you are working from a distance, visualize your client and wait to receive a perception of her body or energy field.

Regardless of where you are, notice what part of her body or field stands out. With the intentions set to clear the source of the problems and a secure connection between your client and her guides (see the section Establishing Alignment in Chapter 5, Anatomy of a Session). Ask where to start. Wait for information to come through either via a vision, a word or sound, or a knowing of what to do. The guides will choose a way to communicate to you that is most effective for you, so whatever information you receive, use your intuition to interpret it. If you are confused, ask a Yes/No question using muscle testing.

At the beginning of the session, I always ask if the core of the client's issue is from a past lifetime. If I get a confirmation, I ask to see that lifetime. For instance, in the following example, I was working with a client who had persistent neck and hip pain.

> *I wait patiently until an image begins to appear. I see a young boy, running through a large field. I see a man on horseback, wielding a spear, chasing the boy. I look at their clothes, at their hair, at the surroundings. I interpret them as being Native American. I wait passively and watch as the scene progresses.*
>
> *I see and feel the boy's fear. He is breathless and terrified. I see the man on horseback, angry, throw the spear. It hits the boy in the back of the neck. The boy crashes to the ground and dies quickly.*

I often begin speaking about the past life story well before I cognitively know what it is. Remaining in an altered state, I receive a glimpse, or a feeling and I begin talking and then the story is interpreted into words from pictures and feelings. One sentence leads to the next and the next, and so on. Feelings are felt. Relationships are understood. Physical experiences are sensed.

HEALING SESSIONS ARE UNIQUE

Each session is different and based entirely on the client's needs at that time. When I fail to fully surrender to the guides and healing team, I begin to see repetition in my work. It could be that I am tired, or it's a day when it's difficult to connect, or there is a fog around my client so I am less able to see what is happening. Regardless, those are the times when the healing session becomes redundant, or even rote.

When we truly surrender our egos and our bodies to become the conduits that we are, magic happens. Being insecure and shy is equally disruptive to the process as being overly assertive and too self-reliant is. Healing in the fourth dimension is a process of surrendering to our higher selves and higher powers. It is a process of being guided so the spiritual healing team can make the necessary changes to the energy of a core issue in the higher dimensions.

It is less important to understand *why* we are doing what we are told, and more important to follow the guidance without hesitation. What we will be told to do will differ each time, but may include the following:

- **Stay exactly where you are, just touching your client's head or shoulders.**
  A lot happens at the head. For one, you may be stabilizing the body, or stabilizing the connection between the body, the mind, the healer (you) and the healing team. Additionally, there are many points on the head that clear different thought processes and emotional issues. And finally, the main centers of the nervous system lie in the cranial and sacral regions and, as in craniosacral therapy, holding the head modulates the balance between the sympathetic and parasympathetic systems, optimizing the function of both. You may choose to look deeper into these healing practices, but even if you don't know exactly how these work and why, it's just as helpful to listen to and follow your intuition about where to place your hands and fingers.

- **Touch a spot on the body with your hands to run energy through organs or acupuncture points along the meridians.**
  If you are already a Reiki practitioner you are familiar with placing your hands on various parts of the body and running energy to corresponding organs and systems. This can be a bit different, however, as the intention is to be of service to the healing team, so you are acting as a conduit for their energy. The team may take over your hands, working through your body. They may send other vibrations of energy besides Reiki, or whatever you have been formally attuned to. Or they may use your arms and hands as the lightning rods that conduct healing work deeper into your client's body.

Foundations of Energy Healing

I often use hand placements to get the energy flowing in the body. Energy can get stuck for many reasons, including trauma, strong emotions, physical pain, illness, stress and more. The body conveys *flow* through sympathetic pulses, subtle pulses in each spot. Just laying the hands on the person will eventually bring the pulse up, however the length of time this takes is different for every person or situation, and can take anywhere from one to five minutes.

When hands are placed apart, say one hand on the shoulder and the other on the wrist, the pulses will, first, come up, second, begin to move alternately (one at a time), and finally, they will move in unison. The unified pulses signal that the flow has been restored and it may be time to move to another position.

Alternatively, you may place your hands on either side of the body, say the abdomen and back, or the top and bottom of a foot. Find the pulses and, first, using your intention, get them to move back and forth between your hands. Second, wait for them to move in sync. At this point you will feel the movement of energy in the client's body between your two hands. Leave your hands in this position for another 10 to 60 seconds and then move to the next position.

- **Touch a spot on the body with one finger, again to run energy through organs or acupuncture points, or to access points deep inside the body.**
Similar to the use of your whole hand, you may be guided to touch spots with one finger for greater accuracy. The finger allows a laser beam of Light to penetrate deeply inside the client's body similar to the Healing Touch Laser technique useful for pain relief and breaking up congestion. However, I have found that with the intention of following the healing team's instructions, "pointing" to one spot directs the energy into cells and molecules to break up and dissolve microscopic issues held at those levels.

Facilitating an Energy Healing Session

- **Brush parts of the aura to stimulate change in the physical body.**
  Often, after the healing team clears or heals trauma or a disruption in the electromagnetic field, I am asked to brush the aura. The movement adds Light and smooth's the field, like putting salve on a cut. Alternatively, just as we as healers are affected by other people's energies, our clients may accumulate the thoughtforms and emotions of places and people they are close to. Gently brushing out the areas of the aura that feel dense or "thick" is a simple way to release them and refresh the energy body. At the very least, this is soothing and will help the client relax. At most, it releases trapped dense and lower vibrations, resulting in the client feeling more positive and optimistic.

- **Send your energy through the client's body to flush out blocks and trapped prana or chi.**
  This technique is very helpful for pain relief. Using your third eye, visualize your client's body, and then move your awareness inside the body. Psychically look or feel for any physical issues or places where the energy seems blocked or tangled. (Obviously this may be new for some of you, and "normal" for others. If this is a novel idea to you, practice with it, and, over time, it will become easier. Studying anatomy is helpful to know where all the organs and glands are, as well as the bones and muscles, etc., to help with visualization.)

  With your intention, breathe your prana into your client's etheric body, into the dense or tangled areas. With your mind, visualize gently releasing and untangling the energy. Allow your imagination to show you how best to do this, as it will be different every time. Take your time, as tangles that have been in place for a long time will need a lot of attention and gentle coaxing to begin to relax. And it may take more than one session to permanently change the blockage.

Of course, you may also be guided to use any of the other techniques you have learned, such as Reiki, Healing Touch,

Craniosacral Therapy, Zero Balancing, hypnotherapy, massage, etc. You were guided to study those techniques in the first place, and your healing team knows you well and will use what comes naturally to you.

During the session, you yourself may experience body movements, such as rocking, gesticulating or stretching. This is the way the body processes the energy moving through you. Additionally, let yourself cough, sneeze or yawn, as it signifies that energy is expanding. Holding those expressions back will thwart the expansion.

You may also find yourself drawn to:

- Tone, either with your voice, a bell or Tibetan or crystal singing bowls.

- Blow over an area of your client's body or breathe out into her etheric field. This is another way to add Light or clear out old energies.

- Hold mudras, which are hands and finger holds that have an effect on the energy of the body.

- Draw or visualize geometric symbols over the body.

Don't be surprised at what comes. And please don't spend too much time questioning it or denying that it is real because that blocks more information from coming in the future.

Above all, please remember: this is a fluid process. Each session is unique. Do what you are guided to do, internally and via the guides, and then, when that task feels complete, ask what is next.

Here is an example of what a typical session with me may look like with a client I will call Lisa:

After spending some time talking about the goals for the session, I have Lisa lie down on a massage table. I place my hands on her shoulders as I psychically scan her body with my eyes closed. I register what is going

on in her etheric and physical bodies by where my
awareness is drawn. In this case, I notice blocked
energy in the second chakra and an absence of energy
in the lower legs or feet.

I then move my eyes up under my eyelids, and
consciously straighten my crown chakra and connect
with my client's guides and any healers who have come
to assist us. I ask them what to focus on first, and wait
to get my instructions. For Lisa, they instruct me to
stay where I am while they begin working on her
second chakra. As the energy begins to clear, I can
sense a deep sadness.

Silently, I ask the guides what this sadness is about.
They begin to show me pictures of a past lifetime in
which Lisa was subservient to her mother. I narrate
out loud what I see in my mind's eye. I continue to
receive pictures, as the story plays out. I also get the
impression that there were other lifetimes when similar
patterns of dominance-subservience occurred. I tell
Lisa all of this.

I feel the impetus to move to Lisa's abdomen, and I
begin to slowly gather and pull out the trauma energy.
As I use my hands in her etheric field, I feel that this
trauma energy is wrapped around her organs with
what seems like tentacles, so I visualize gently unwrap-
ping them and pulling them out. When that feels
complete, I muscle-test whether or not I am correct,
and I get a Yes response.

I wait for my next instructions. My attention is pulled
to Lisa's lower legs and feet, and I can feel that Lisa's
energy is not filling that part of her body. I move to the
foot of the table, place my hands on the backs of her
ankles, and wait patiently for the pulses there to sync.
While waiting, I psychically scan her body to see where
her energy lies. I psychically see an image of Lisa,
scared and protective of herself, standing above her
right shoulder. Silently, I speak to her with soothing
words: "It's okay. You are safe. Come back in."
I wait patiently until I see her energy move back into
her body. I place my hands lightly on Lisa's feet. I
watch Lisa breathe and I feel the flow of energy. I wait
until I feel the energy travel up her body on the
inhalation, and fill her feet on the exhalation. When

*that feels complete, I ask for my next set of instruc-
tions.*

*I see an image in my mind's eye of a series of points on
Lisa's head. I understand that these points are from the
Access Bars therapy. (Access Bars is an energy
technique taught by teachers trained through the
Access Consciousness programs.) The points I see
connect to the issues of healing, joy, sadness and the
body. I understand immediately that these points will
contribute to the release of these past life issues for
Lisa. I move to sit at her head, and place my fingers on
these points.*

*While I do this, I scan her body again. I also ask the
guides if there is anything else they would like me to do.
I watch as energy in her etheric field is cleared and
manipulated by the healing team.*

*I continue on, in this way, until I feel the energy
subsiding. When I do, I ask the healing team if they are
complete. I hold space for Lisa until I get a clear feeling
that we are complete.*

This kind of session typically takes one hour. When the session is
finished, Lisa feels calm, relaxed and clear. She reports that
understanding her history with her mother, and having it
identified as dominant/subservient, will help her break the
behavior patterns. Over time, Lisa becomes less fearful overall
and able to stay grounded in her body. She is capable of creating
appropriate boundaries and stating her needs and that allows her
to maintain the power balance with her mother.

Facilitating an Energy Healing Session

HOME PRACTICE

Surrender to the flow of ideas and information, even if you are not one-hundred percent sure why you are doing what you are doing, and all will be perfect. When in doubt, fall back on your training: Reiki, Seichim, Sekhem, Karuna, Access Bars, massage, Theta Healing, Resonance Repatterning… whatever you have been trained to do.

Unless you are professionally licensed, do not diagnose or offer nutritional or pharmaceutical advice. Stay within the guidelines of your local medical laws.

THE HEALING TEAM AT WORK

I received a craniosacral therapy session for a minor back injury recently, during which I could see a male spirit standing next to my therapist. She continued to place her hands on the various parts of my body that were appropriate for her work. And at the same time I "watched" this spirit (via my third eye) place crystals on each of my hips and then on my heart. He then somehow psychically activated those crystals. Before long a trauma memory came back to me and I had a great emotional release. The therapist said she could feel energetic shifts in my heart center.

While you are holding space, moving energy and communicating with your client, your healing team is working on the big picture on the etheric level and in the various dimensions. Each session can vacillate between being very busy for you—moving around, receiving psychic information, adjusting the body—to being very quiet for you while the guides do most of the work. And the more

91

you expect them and invite them in, the more they will be apparent to you.

As a quantum energy healer, you are most effective when you drop your thoughts about what to do and open into pure guidance. This is true no matter what kind of healing methods and techniques you are trained in. At some point it is best to put down what you "know" and surrender into Trust.

Below I list some of the many things I have witnessed the healing team do. This is a small list of an *infinite* number of healing, altering, preparing and loving energies they offer. What I describe below are the ways I have learned to interpret and describe the sensations I receive based on my training and intuition. As always, this is information that comes in through my psychic filter, presented in the way that best allows for my understanding. It is appropriate that you may experience and interpret the information differently based on your unique filter and experiences.

- **Creating electrical changes in the body**
  One of the first times I saw this was when working on a man who, years ago, had a traumatic brain injury. The healing team began rewiring his brain and nervous system—actually using tiny tools inside his brain and brainstem and then in various places in his spine. My client could feel it, and experienced clearer thinking and reasoning afterwards.

- **Rewiring molecules, cells and DNA**
  I have witnessed the spiritual healing team clearing out karmic and genetic ties to illness by working deep within cells and molecules. This feels like tiny beings or tiny instruments of Light operating deep inside the muscles. I clairvoyantly see the cells popping and exploding into tiny bursts of Light.

  Similarly, the healing team can clean and clear any illness or behavior patterns that we hold in our DNA from our many lifetimes. These patterns may be karmic or genetic. Karma is accumulated through our own lifetimes or the experiences of our families, or society. Genetic patterns exist in our biology, and have been handed down through our family lines. DNA work is very subtle, and I often know it is happening via claircognizance, rather than feel or see it.

- **Clearing the energy grid**
  Our bodies exist as part of a huge grid of energy that organizes life as we know it. There is no difference between your body, the energy outside it, and the energy inside it, other than the way the energy expresses itself—the *form*. Indeed, the energy that is on the outside *is* the energy that is on the inside.

The grid is energy, pure Light and Intelligence. The grid holds and is comprised of the different forms that the energy is separated into so that this 3-D world is one hundred percent believable to the five senses. It holds the etheric blueprints and energy bodies for every creation on the planet. It anchors your soul to your body. And it also anchors your body to the planet and all its inhabitants, because there is no beginning and no ending to the grid.

It literally looks like a grid, with lines of Light connected by crystals of Light. I often perceive the grid as being made of pink light. Many times, before I had ever heard of the grid, the spiritual healing team had me draw lines over my clients' bodies with my fingertips. I would draw a line, for instance, across the hips. I would repeat this three times, and then I would be called to draw lines straight down the legs, three times. The lines I was impelled to draw always connected to each other in either a rectangular or triangular shape, following the lines of the body or the connections to the chakras. As I came to understand the fifth-dimensional meridians, I saw the correlations between my "outlines" and that meridian system.

The energy of the Grid is creation energy. And it is completely malleable. The way to transform the energy of everything you put into your body is through peaceful, loving contemplation. So in 4th dimensional healing, even without changing the physical matter of a substance, you can change the energy that comprises the matter though your loving intention.

Foundations of Energy Healing

- **Sending in Love and Light**
  Sometimes clients just need to be soothed or made to feel
  safe. In their unconditional Love for us, the healing team
  brings in beautiful iridescent pink and gold Light to fill their
  fields. This Light expands (potentially infinitely), bathing the
  client in a blanket of Love.

  We can call on the Archangels to do this after clearing a
  trauma or entity from the field with the following invocation:

  *Gabriel, please fill all voids with crystal white light. Chamuel, add pink
  love light. Raphael, send green healing light. Zadkiel, pour forth violet
  rays of transmutation. Jophiel, send sunshine yellow rays of illumination.
  Uriel, please send ruby-gold. And Michael, seal this healing with your
  blue light.*

- **Sending negative energy to the higher dimensions to be
  transmuted back into Light and then returned to the
  body**
  Many people carry a constant supply of fear and anger in their
  bodies and minds. In the past few decades, many therapies
  have been developed to process and work through these
  feelings. Each one of them has its place, yet too often,
  processing no longer serves one's highest good.

  In 4th-dimensional healing, the healing team is capable of
  releasing all negative feelings that no longer serve the
  individual. They do this by lifting lower-density emotional
  charges into the higher dimensions and easily transmute them
  back into Light. The Light is then returned to the energy
  field. (To me, this looks and feels like clouds of condensed
  energy being carried out of the body and into the farthest
  reaches of the energy field, and then raining down in beautiful
  gold flecks.)

- **Reprogramming Lightcodes**
  Lightcodes are embedded codes of information connected to
  the grid. Along the lines of a computer programming
  language (although infinitely more detailed), they define each
  person's personality, experiences, perspectives, health, body
  type, history, etc. Lightcodes are the building blocks that

create the separate blueprint of each individual.

Lightcodes look like ribbons of energy, decorated with disks with different kinds of symbols on them, of which there are an infinite number of patterns. There are mental, emotional, and physical lightcodes. Some lightcodes symbolize belief systems, while others pertain to organs and systems in the body.

The energy that makes up Who We Are is fluid. It is both receptive to, and the co-creator of, our environment and activities. This energy is malleable and moveable. Therefore, we can ask for changes in the lightcodes. For instance, if someone is living with a chronic illness it is likely that it is from genetic or karmic coding. We can request that this coding be revised or changed or deleted. Alternately, the healing team may tell us when it is time to change or add codes.

One of the ways I have experienced this is as follows: the healing team tells me to hold out my hand. They hand me a disk and give me instructions about where to place it in my client's field. After I have done this, the client notices (over time) that the old issues shift and new ways of being manifest.

When the healing team activates the lightcodes, in effect they alter patterns so they are more in accordance with each person's Higher Self. It is like pointing someone in the right direction again.

- **Grounding**
Fear and anxiety cause people to "leave their bodies." This is a bit more literal than you might think: parts of the soul, or *soul fragments*, lift away from the physical body to try to feel safer because the soul does not want to have the experience that the body is having. Paradoxically, this causes more fear and anxiety.

Energetically, you may be able to see your client's energy imprint outside of the body, often to the side, but sometimes floating above. You may be able to feel this when you are at the client's feet, as little or no energy will flow in the legs and feet.

The healing team can help the client ground by sending Earth energy up into the field. This feels something like the client being planted into the Earth, and vine-like energy moving up the legs and torso. The healing team can also create a safe enough space for the client that the soul fragments agree to "move back in."

- **Expanding**
  Much like you would stretch your body when your muscles are tight, the healing team has the ability to stretch the energy bodies to allow them to expand. This opens the client up to new information and opportunities. I don't know how else to describe it, other than to say it feels like a relief... like being able to take a massive deep breath. This quiets the mind and floods the room with feelings of joy and peace.

Following is an excerpt of my narration of a partial healing session on Tammi. As the session was conducted over the phone, the healing team did all of the work on her, while giving me the visualizations, sensations and information Tammi needed to process the session.

The intentions that Tammi set for the session were as follows:

- To balance and organize time and energy between her doctorate thesis, daily exercise and growth opportunities at work;

- To continue to work on opening her third eye;

- To create motivation to be more productive; and

- To clear triangulation energy between her, her husband and his mother.

Facilitating an Energy Healing Session

What follows is the transcription of the recording of the session:

I feel the healing team is coming in and doing a sweep of the body, assessing where in the body there is holding. They begin working mostly on the muscles of the shoulder and chest and the throat.

And this energy, this tightness here, is related to fear that has been accumulating behind the heart. So the energy is moving in and around the heart.

And as that energy moves out, I yawn and take deep breaths, as tension is being released in the jaw and shoulders.

This tension has to do with the sense of overwhelm, which is a mindset, it's not the reality, but just a mindset... it is from the fear that you will be over-whelmed. All of this has to do with prior school, classes, and learning a language... feeling overwhelmed in one class or another as if there is not enough time... and because of the language barrier there is confusion. And that your mind was working two ways at one time: translating and then actually producing the work. And this created a block from the fear around the amount of work that this was.

I feel the energy moving through the body. I'm feeling it really settling in the belly.

And so the team is recognizing how much of this fear needs to be held onto and how much can be released as part of your past.

And what the healing team is doing now is they are taking the trauma out of those memories. They are removing the trauma. Pulling it out of the right side of the jaw.

We're yawning again as it is clearing.

And your middle back is relaxing. And as this is released in the body, the message I am getting is that your mind will be able to make more sense of things.

Your mind will be less affected and afraid and confused.

And this is where the organization comes in. And the way I feel it is that your energy is coming into alignment.

And the way I feel that is through my torso - energy is lining up and settling and grounding. So there is a quieting of the system. And they are instilling in the body a desire to move and exercise and swim, so that you will feel that in the morning when you wake up. I feel my legs are energized. There is a "knowing" that is coming into your energy field. This is an understanding that, "Of course this is what I'm going to do. Of course this would be best for me." And there is an alignment around that knowing. It is a very strong solid connection.

And energy is being cleared out of the abdomen and gut. I see that it is a past lifetime issue.
This energy is the fear of not being able to take care of yourself, and not having the resources to do so in other lifetimes. This is (an unconscious) memory of not having the resources... And the way it presents itself today is as a part of the excuse not to get up early. This is the way that the mind works with subconscious memory. It says, "I'm tired. I don't have time." This is what the mind says, and it pulls up that memory of, "Oh, well, I really can't take care of myself anyway." And the healing team is lifting that out of the gut now, as well as the abdomen, the solar plexus....

The session continues this way for about an hour. I am clear that it is finished when I feel all energies subside. I always double-check with the healing team, asking if they are complete before I remove myself from the client's energy field. Afterwards, Tammi reported that she could feel a lot of the movement and changes occurring within her body as I worked.

I also facilitate healings from a distance without verbal contact with the client. To do this, I move into a meditative state and create my connections with the client, her guides and the healing team. I hold space while the healing unfolds in my mind's eye. The sessions run similarly to in-person and phone sessions, again, taking about an hour. When they are finished, generally I email notes from the session to the client.

I have noticed that, over time, clients feel a progressive relief in their physical, mental and emotional symptoms. Thus they are able to react to life events differently, staying present to what unfolds rather than repeating past habits and patterns.

HOME PRACTICE

Mental relaxation is the key to working with your healing team. Keep checking in with them, but if you are not receiving clear information, relinquish all control and allow your hands to move themselves. It is not necessary for you to know or understand everything. In fact, most of a 4th-dimensional healing session happens within a cloak of the mystery.

Set the intention that you are lovingly holding space and you are the conduit of the energies moving from the spiritual healing team through you, and trust that it is all happening as it should be.

FYI, I have been known to tell my clients, "The healing team was working at a really high vibration. I am unclear about what they were doing, but it felt great." My clients are perfectly content to hear that!

---

7. Clearing Trauma

What if every disease known to man
was really just a physical manifestation of the illusion
that we are separate from Source?

Removing trauma is often a big part of an energy healing session. Mental and emotional trauma is often veiled or hidden, manifesting as chronic illness or emotional pain. Most people are not in touch with what exactly the core of their suffering is, and so they are not able to find relief through traditional forms of healthcare.

Ayurveda (translated from Sanskrit, meaning Life Knowledge) is the ancient Indian medical system that teaches that illness and disease are the result of the illusion of separation from Source. All suffering stems from this illusion that we are alone here on the planet, and that life is dangerous. Of course, it is impossible to actually be separated from Source, though life as we have known it on this planet has been a trial of separation, where the feelings and beliefs that we are alone seem real and powerful.

There are many causes of trauma—from suffering at the hands of a culture or society, to survival issues, such as starvation and illness, from the death of loved ones, to being victimized or even from being a perpetrator of a crime. Anything that causes fear and its complementary emotions (anxiety, panic, worry, guilt, grief, loneliness, confusion, and so on) causes suffering. These emotions, which begin in the mental and emotional bodies, create blocks in our energy, eventually manifesting as a physical illness.

If we really knew that we weren't alone, if we knew of our power and connection to Source, we would never be afraid, never doubt who and what and where we were. We would be in a perpetual dance of conscious co-creation with, and surrender to, our Divine Selves. All our energy bodies and systems would be in perfect harmony, creating a state of vibrant health.

In many lifetimes, trauma may be the result of a soul contract to have a certain kind of experience, perhaps to survive beyond the physical confines of a healthy body, to give up or forget one's power, or to love through loss. Each experience offers life lessons and opportunities for compassion.

Once manifested, trauma may become *karmic*, meaning that it may repeat itself throughout lifetimes over and over again. The persistence of suffering over time confirms the belief that one is a victim of random incidents and situations. In fact, trauma and the resulting suffering may be clues that the belief in the illusion of separation still exists.

Every soul's journey—be it in a day, a lifetime, or multiple lifetimes—is to travel away from Source only, ultimately, to return to Source. Imagine you are holding a dog on a retractable leash. The leash allows the dog to venture out away from you without being disconnected from you. The dog may only go one foot, two feet...even farther. The dog can only go so far but you *ALWAYS* hold him safely. So too do we spiritual beings travel away from Source—and the farther we go the more pain we may experience —without ever being disconnected.

Trauma is also *attractive*, meaning that the vibration of trauma keeps attracting more of the same. Additionally, the vibration of that belief that you will continue to suffer attracts more experiences that will be felt as suffering. Retraining the mind and emotions to reframe experiences can be extremely beneficial to begin to turn this around.

One of the ways energy healing is beneficial is that the healing team is quite capable of releasing trauma held in the physical body, as well as any of the energy bodies. In the past, the way to release trauma was to consciously work through our emotions and memories. More recently, as humanity has evolved, it is less important to work through the mental process of understanding the pain and the emotional process of feeling the feelings again, and instead, just release the dense energy.

In the early stages of healing, there is much clearing of karmic ties and emotional attachments to trauma energy, as well as the physical manifestations of it in the body. As the healings progress over time, more light can enter the energy field, soul fragments may return, and clients become more and more peaceful for longer periods of time.

ABUSE

Abuse occurs physically, emotionally, verbally and sexually.

Abuse can occur in childhood or in adulthood. The effects of abuse may be held as imprints on any level of the astral bodies. Imprints are beliefs that have been created due to a heightened emotional response. Emotional responses in general may be positive or negative. However, in the case of trauma, they are negative.

What may seem like an innocuous incident to one person may actually be the worst kind of abuse to another. The experience of abuse, and the resulting traumatic energy signature is extremely individual. As a healer, keep in mind that it is the experience or the interpretation of the client that has led to the energetic issue, not how you might have responded under the same circumstances. In other words, do not minimize what another has interpreted as traumatic just because it doesn't "seem like a big deal" to you.

In the mental body, imprints are held as false beliefs about yourself or the world. In the emotional body, imprints are held as fear, and the complementary emotions. In the etheric body imprints block the flow of life-force energy. And in the physical body, imprints manifest as pain and illness.

Sexual abuse comes up often and is not to be shied away from. Studies show that two-thirds of girls in this country have been sexually abused. The same may be seen for boys; however sexual abuse of boys appears to be commonly underreported, under-recognized, and undertreated.

Sexual abuse in males may even come in the form of society or family patterns leading to exhibiting abusive behavior. In this way, men can be taught that abuse is normal or expected from them.

As we clear the energetic and karmic patterns of abuse from victims, we create fewer perpetrators in the future.

If someone tells you that she has been abused, sexually or otherwise, it is completely unprofessional to respond in any way that shows you are shocked, scared, judgmental, or questioning. I have had clients, and I have heard of others, who, when telling their therapist that they were victims of incest, were asked, "Are you sure you aren't making that up?" There is nothing more devastating to a person who has been made to keep a horrible secret her whole life than being accused of lying by her trusted therapist.

Be gentle about talking about what you see or realize. For instance, if you see sexual abuse and feel the resulting emotional responses, understand that the client may not be consciously aware of it and your expressing it bluntly may break rapport or cause unnecessary trauma. Remember that in quantum energy healing, knowing the "why" may be interesting, but is not necessary.

Abuse can cause vicarious trauma in the healer, meaning it can trigger the healer's own fears. When you are in close contact with your client, you move into resonance with her. This is due to the fact that in healing, resonance means the two of you will begin to vibrate at frequencies in accordance with each other. This opens up intimate levels of communication. The result of this is that you will pick up on issues that may be hidden from your client's consciousness, or that are hidden from public information.

Clearing Trauma

If you are triggered by what you see, understand that the emotions or energy have hit a place in you that resonates at the same frequency. You will draw into your practice those individuals who have similar traumas to be cleared. If you need to work on your self-esteem, for example, clients who need the same will be drawn to your vibration. Begin to notice the similarities in your clients and you will see a clearer picture of yourself. The reason behind this is simple: as my first Reiki teacher used to say, "Give a healing, get a healing."

If you are not used to clearing your own trauma by yourself, please find someone to help you do that. As proven with your clients, it's often helpful to have a safe place in which to heal with another person who can witness your journey in a loving way.

If you are feeling sensations or emotions during the session, and you are not clear about where they are coming from, ask the question: *Is this mine or hers or ours?* Be careful not to take on what is not yours to be cleared. Do not use your body to relieve someone else of his pain, even though your empathy might make it seem like the right thing to do. That might demonstrate a lack of appropriate boundaries.

We are in charge of our own energy fields. We are in charge of what comes in and what goes out. In the case of healing, a certain amount of resonance is desired because it allows us to create comprehension and compassion. Those emotions are used to provide us with pertinent information for healing, and not for sympathy. Sympathy can result in our agreeing (usually unconsciously) to take the clients' pain from them. Taking that on, and making ourselves sick in the process, is completely unproductive and is *not* healing.

Better yet, if you are aware that you share the same issue, you might consider asking the guides and healing team to include you in the healing session.

PAST LIVES

I have been conducting past life regressions since 2003. In these sessions, I have witnessed hundreds of people gaining clarity, clearing patterns, and healing emotionally and physically through this process.

The soul divides into twelve aspects at a time, each living concurrently in different historical time periods and at different locations. This is possible because time is not the linear construct we believe it to be. All time exists simultaneously, but we cannot see that because the concept of linear time allows us to map a course of historical change... a much-needed paradigm on this planet for us to perpetuate belief in our separate lives.

So, really, *past* life regressions are actually *other* or *concurrent* life regressions. They are a glimpse into some of the emotional issues our souls are trying to work through at the same time. And, if a soul cannot work out that issue in one lifetime through one personality, it carries that over to another personality. The beauty of past life regression work is that, as we heal one aspect, we heal the others. As we clear a fear from our own lifetime, we potentially heal the same fear in any other lifetime that we are experiencing it, and vice versa.

I have seen a few regressions that can be traced to the time and the place where the story occurred. This is my favorite one:

Dean was about to take a vacation with his wife where he would be flying to a distant island. He hadn't been on a plane in years because of a fear of flying. He came to me asking to do a past life regression to see if his fear had roots from any experience from a previous lifetime.

During his past life regression, Dean relived a lifetime where he was an insurance salesman in Pennsylvania in the mid-50s. He left his family to fly to Ohio on business. He could see a name and logo on the napkin that was served to him with his drink; an airline no longer in existence. He had a strong memory of the sound of the engine as it began to fail. He felt the plane jerk, shudder, and finally careen out of the sky to the ground, where he died.

After his session, Dean went home and searched on the internet to see what he could find. Lo and behold, he found references to a small airline that flew in the 50s between Pennsylvania and Ohio, and saw that the insignia was the same as the one he had seen on his napkin in his regression. He also found a newspaper article citing a crash that sounded exactly like the one that came from his memory.

Had Dean actually been on that airplane or was he dredging up old fears coming from an article that he may have read in *National Geographic* in third grade? The answer is: it doesn't matter. A few weeks after his session, he successfully boarded the plane to the island with his wife, and had a great, stress-free vacation.

I cannot prove that past lives exist for us. And if this idea of multiple lifetimes does not suit you, then scrap it. You do not need it to do healing work. You, like a healer friend of mine, might prefer to think of this work as clearing issues from cellular memory or genetic coding. It matters not, because the intention to remove trauma energy is all that is important.

8. Self-Care

What if our ability to help someone else heal
was dependent upon our doing
our own healing work as well?

Everyone gets challenged sometimes. And those of us who are healers are more likely to be sensitive to our environment, and to experience deep emotions that can throw us off for days. For these reasons, it is important to learn how to take care of ourselves energetically and emotionally. In fact, it is necessary to develop a personal practice for our own health and healing in order to stay well and balanced as we offer our services to others.

Lightworkers often incarnate carrying the energies of innocence and hope, a naiveté. That, accompanied with an often very high vibration, potentially sets us up for extreme pain when we are confronted by the heavier energies of this planet. As each soul has to move through its own karmic growth over lifetimes on this planet, healers, too, carry their own traumas and wounds from past lifetimes into this one.

We all hold archetypal patterns in our energy fields. Archetypes are defined in Jungian psychology as collectively inherited unconscious ideas, patterns of thought, images, etc., universally present in individual psyches. They are descriptions of personality types that are mutually understandable by all. Some of the common archetypes for those who do healing work include the Wounded Healer, the Caregiver, the Warrior, and the Innocent.

Foundations of Energy Healing

ARCHETYPES

The **Wounded Healer** is one who is initiated into the art of healing through some form of personal hardship—anything from an actual physical injury or illness to the loss of all of one's earthly possessions. Regardless of the kind of wound, the challenge inherent in this archetype is that one finds oneself unable to turn to others for help beyond a certain degree of support.[1]

As the Wounded Healer, one pushes oneself to consciously experience and go through one's wounds in an effort to receive their blessings. The Wounded Healer consistently revisits the painful new places in himself where the wound is leading, so he can allow himself to be re-created by the wound. This is often a positive growth experience, allowing the old self to "die" in the process, while a new, more expansive and empowered part is potentially born.

The negative—or shadow—aspect of the Wounded Healer is the addiction to the familiar pain of the wounds. This addiction is a compelling sense of pain, and one eschews relief. One never allows oneself to be out of crisis or to feel happy. Over the years, I have known many psychics and healers who have been sickly or obese, who take on the wounds of the world and live dysfunctional lives themselves.

The **Caregiver** archetype may be closely related to the role of the Wounded Healer. The Caregiver is one who feels that she receives love through selfless acts towards others. She is proficient at putting herself second if it means helping another person receive the attention he needs. (Envision the stereotypical selfless mother or grandmother).

The wounded side of the Caregiver has no boundaries, fearing that she will be considered selfish if she says, "No." Unable to feel whole within herself, she loses herself in the caring of everyone else.

The positive aspects of the **Warrior** archetype include physical strength and the ability to protect, defend, and fight for one's rights. Characteristics such as invincibility and loyalty, virility, physical power and toughness of will are all aspects of this archetype, as well as being unbreakable and fighting to the death.

The wound the Warrior carries with him is the pain of facing selfish, evil thieves and killers who embody our worst nightmares of lawlessness and unchecked male dominance.[2] Wounded Warriors are quick to rise to the challenge, yet internally exhausted and, sometimes, even broken. (Think *Buffy the Vampire Slayer.*) They often have hair-triggers and are quick to distrust others.

The archetype of the **Innocent (or Divine Child)** may have been personified by Anne Frank, who wrote in her diary that in spite of all the horror surrounding her family while hiding from Nazis in an attic in Amsterdam, she still believed that humanity was basically good. The Divine Child is associated with innocence, purity, and redemption.[3]

The shadow energy of the Innocent manifests in pessimism and depression, or as the absence of the possibility of miracles and of the transformation of evil to good. Hopelessness may set in and with it, powerlessness. We are unable to defend ourselves against negative forces.

SELF-HEALING TOOLS

Our objective with quantum energy healing is to release and relinquish our wounds and traumas, thereby allowing the depth of holistic healing to take place. It does not serve us to perpetually remain in the wounded aspect of whatever archetypal patterns we hold. So, with the goal of lightening our burdens, we must face our demons and embrace our own healing.

Some of the simplest tried-and-true, self-help practices include journaling and moving our bodies via exercise or any other kind of self-expressive movement.

Journaling is a great stress reducer because it allows us to take the time we need to sort a situation out and come up with conclusions for moving forward. It works both the left and right sides of the brain simultaneously. In this way, the conscious mind processes the thoughts and information at hand, while the subconscious mind is able to calm itself through visualizing and conceptualizing the same issues.

Either starting a morning journaling practice, or merely journaling as needed, is a highly effective way to provide us with the time and space necessary to relax and find positive ways to move forward. Additionally, we can begin our day in the most positive light by establishing a morning practice of journaling gratitude statements, goals for the day, or setting our intentions for short segments of the day—what Abraham-Hicks calls *Segment Intending*. But guard against making this a "to-do list." Allow expression and creativity instead of merely listing the tasks for the day.

Finding ways to move the body helps to release emotions stuck in the limbic brain. The limbic brain governs our survival, and so our fears are processed through this part of the brain, stimulating the hypothalamus, which sets off a complex series of events: the stress response. The hypothalamus is found at the base of the brain just above the pituitary gland. It acts as the link between the nervous system and the endocrine (hormonal) system by monitoring many of the body's internal conditions and releasing hormones. When the hypothalamus gets activated due to stress, it signals the pituitary and adrenal glands to release various hormones related to stress and survival (aka, the fight-or-flight response), including cortisol and adrenaline. These hormones ready the body for defense, either fighting or running.

The best way to stop the flow of these hormones and calm the body down is through movement. In the wild, animals that have been threatened or shocked have the same fight-or-flight response we do, but unlike us, they instinctively know to "shake it off" afterwards. Quite literally, an animal that tends to freeze or play dead when under attack will, after returning to safety, shake from the head to the tail to re-set its system. The difference for us is that we are not usually physically threatened, even though the body instinctively responds as if we are.

Please note: a thought or image creates the same response, whether it is from an actual occurrence or an imaginary one. The subconscious mind cannot discern between "real" and "imaginary." Your thoughts create real physical responses, no matter where they come from.

Finding a fun and comfortable kind of movement, such as dancing, taking a walk in nature or attending a yoga class, can help you recover from the toxic results of stressful thoughts. Deep breathing is a natural by-product of movement and exercise, and interrupts the stress response cycle. Slow, deep breathing signals the brain that the threat has passed, and all systems can return to normal. We can feel the muscles in our back, neck and extremities soften and relax when the breath deepens. In fact, each exhalation allows more and more adrenaline to be cleared from the body and reinvigorates the muscles.

Most kinds of slow or repetitive movement help the mind return its awareness to the body and its connection to the Earth. Dance is a wonderful way to allow the body any movement that it may desire in order to release muscle tension. At times, loud music with powerful beats will be conducive to release, while at other times slow, quiet or meditative movement will be more helpful.

Allowing our bodies (and spirits) to lead the way is therapeutic in itself, because so often throughout our lifetimes, others impose their will upon us rather than our being allowed to follow our own inner guidance. It is healing to be attentive to our own needs, regardless of what we have been programmed to think is the "right" or expected way to do things.

Walking outside when possible, breathing the fresh air into the lungs, smelling the scents and fragrances that soothe the mind, and allowing the colors of nature to stimulate the irises in the eyes, quiet the stress response. Feeling our feet on the Earth helps us to ground into the body and feel more peaceful. The whole process allows the mind to quiet and be more creative, forming new decisions and new ways of looking at a situation.

Meditative movement classes like yoga, tai chi and qi gong create the same result. These practices focus on staying present and "in the moment," instead of fearing the future and/or regretting the past. Being present lets us concentrate on what is actually happening, creating a quietness and focus that automatically stops the mental and physical results of the fight-or-flight response. These practices also balance all the systems in the body, creating a sense of ease and grace.

Finally, it is always appropriate to ask our own spiritual healing teams to help. Remember, they will not intervene unless asked. Personally, I request healing at night, when I first lie down to go to sleep. As much as possible, I tell them what I would like to work on. As with your clients, the clearer the intentions, the more the spiritual healing team can and will help.

On occasions when I have felt stuck or scared or anxious, I have told my healing team that very thing and asked them for help releasing the old feelings. At other times, I have asked them to help me progress to the next level, however that may occur. And again at other times, I have told them something specific that I want, and asked them to help me manifest it. The results of these sessions, as true with any 4th-dimensional healing sessions, are multifaceted, offering any combination of physical, mental and emotional relief, as well as new ideas, opportunities and challenges. I keep in mind that these are all the steps necessary for progress.

For those who choose a path of healing, no matter if via a conventional Western medical career or an alternative healing practice, it is imperative to keep your body, mind and energy field clear and balanced. Developing a self-healing and self-help program is vital to your growth—and health—as a healer.

Self-Care

In the chapters that follow, I describe meditations and visualizations designed to help keep your energy clear, your body grounded and your mind peaceful.

ENDNOTES: CHAPTER 8

1. Carolyn Myss, "A Gallery of Archetypes," www.myss.com/library/contracts/three_archs.asp, (2010, Myss.com).

2. Ibid.

3. Ibid.

9. Mind-Body Practices

*What if we knew that quieting our minds would open
hidden channels of communication with our bodies,
allowing healing at every level?*

Following is a series of guided meditations designed to help you stay self-aware with a clear mind and calm body. They will help you bring the information in the previous chapters into practice, giving you first-hand awareness of the energies that lie within and around your physical body. You may also choose to use them with clients, of course.

Foundations of Energy Healing

BODY AWARENESS EXERCISE

This Body Awareness Exercise brings you into intimate contact with your physical self. As you watch your breath, you can begin to see the quality of the energy within and around your body. You may even notice the chakras and the aura. Or you may experience your body merge with the energy around you. The possibilities are limitless.

On an emotional level you may see and feel the changes as you move through the different areas of your body, for example, your abdomen may feel open and receptive to the breath, while your chest may be more constricted. Strengthen the wisdom body (*vijnanamaya kosha*) through your level of concentration and focus. Enhance the bliss body (*anandamaya kosha*) by the radiance emanating from your heart.

Whatever your experience, do not judge or define it in any way. Practice being mindfully aware of what you notice. You may choose to record this visualization for ease of practice or access the following online at randibotnick.com/listeninglibrary.

Allow your body to completely relax... Inhale and feel the breath flow from the soles of your feet to the crown of your head, like a gentle slow motion wave. With each exhalation, allow tension to flow out of your body... Bring your awareness to the fingers of the left hand. Inhale breath and awareness through the fingers and up your left arm... Exhale, release your arm into the support of the Earth... Feel your entire arm, hand and fingers now. Experience the sensations... there may be lightness or heaviness, warmth or coolness, tingling or energy. Allow your sense of relaxation to deepen with each exhalation.

Now bring your awareness to your fingertips of your right hand and inhale the breath up your arm, exhale and completely relax. As you relax your arms, become

*more aware of your feelings and sensations... Notice
any difference between your two arms. Focus all of
your awareness on your sensations and then relax into
them.*

*Now bring your awareness down to the toes of your left
foot, drawing the wave of your breath up to the top of
your leg... And on exhalation, relax the leg fully... feel
and see the breath in your foot, ankle, lower leg, knee,
all the way up to the top of your thigh...*

*Now bring your awareness into your right leg. Allow
the wave of breath to flow up the right leg... and with
the exhalation, completely surrender the weight of your
leg... Feel and see both legs now and with each breath,
become more aware of all the sensations in your legs...
Notice any difference between the two legs... With each
exhalation, relax even more deeply... Listen to the
sound as the waves of your breath roll through your
body.*

*Now bring the breath and your awareness up into the
hips, pelvis and buttocks. Notice the areas where your
awareness and breath enter easily and those that are
less accessible... On the inhalation, feel your pelvic
area naturally expand... and exhaling, allow it to rest
down into the earth... With each inhalation, feel the
pelvic floor being drawn gently up into the abdomen
and with each exhalation, allow it to completely
release... feel the wave of breath rising up from the
pelvis filling the abdomen...*

*Feel the abdomen rise and fall. Explore the abdomen
with your awareness... With each exhalation, the
abdomen becomes softer and softer. Feel the softness
touch the lower back. Explore the sensations in the low
back and allow this area to soften into the earth.*

*Now allow your breath and awareness to flow up your
spine... With each inhalation, the spine fills with
sensation.... With each exhalation, the spine relaxes*

into the earth... feeling your breath now through the entire back... Inhaling, sensing; exhaling, completely relaxing.

Now bring your awareness again to the rising and falling of your abdomen... As you inhale, draw the breath up into the solar plexus, feeling that area fully with your breath and awareness... as you exhale, relax into the center of that awareness... Now focus the breath up into your heart and lungs, and with each exhalation, relax deeper and deeper into the center of your heart. Notice areas of tightness or openness, lightness or heaviness as you explore the chest...

Draw breath into your neck and throat... Exhale, allowing any attention to be released... Allow the breath to flow up through your head... and with each inhalation, become more aware of the sensations... With each exhalation, relax... Relax your jaw... your eyes... your forehead and the back of your head... soften your inner ears... and relax into the earth.

And the body as a whole now... Notice where your awareness is naturally drawn within the body... explore the body freely noticing all the feelings and sensations... Feel the breath touching every part of your body...

Feel your entire body now washed by the gentle waves of breath, from the soles of your feet and the tips of your fingers all the way to the crown of your head... Feel the peace and complete relaxation as your breathing becomes softer and softer... Feel the sensations in your body becoming softer... more subtle... Relax into them.

Notice, where does your body begin and where does it end?

(Pause.)

Now allow the waves of your breath to be felt a little more strongly, rising up through the soles of your feet, and rising and falling in the abdomen... As the breath becomes stronger, allow the sensations in the body to increase... As you are ready, begin to gently move your fingers and toes. Stretch and move any way that feels good. And over the next few breaths, gently open your eyes.

CHAKRA BALANCE

The following guided meditation is best used by recording it in your own voice and then listening to it with your eyes closed. Or access the following online at randibotnick.com/listeninglibrary.

Sit in a comfortable position or lie down on your back keeping your spine straight. Breathe slowly and deeply for a few minutes, settling into your body with a quiet mind.

Imagine a beautiful, iridescent light wrapping around your body from under your feet to above your head. These strands of light soothe your energy body, forming an egg shape around you, sealing you in a beautiful cocoon. This cocoon allows you to feel even more relaxed and very safe.

Imagine energy entering through the back of the third chakra, behind your solar plexus, to clear any stuck or stagnant places. The back of the third chakra governs the energy of motivation. It gives you the ability to move forward with good self-esteem and healthy ego strength.

121

*As the back of the third chakra clears, the energy flows
through to the front of the third chakra. The energy of
the front of the third chakra helps you with setting
healthy boundaries. You may notice that it becomes
easier to breathe. Picture the chakra starting to look
like an open tube that allows for more relaxed
emotions, where feelings, thoughts and beliefs are no
longer able to get stuck in the body.*

*Follow the energy down to the front of the second
chakra next, releasing any fear and guilt that are a
result of your desires. As this clears, the energy flows
into the back of the second chakra. Feel your sacrum
relax. The energy in the back of the second chakra
fuels your ability to step forward into the world to do
your work or fulfill your passions.*
*Follow the energy down to the root chakra next, which
"faces" down between your legs. Feel the energy pour
into your hips and rain down your legs, forming a tube
around your legs that connects to the Earth's energies,
allowing the Earth to feed your field. This "food" from
the Earth is healing, soothing, informative, nurturing,
and sustaining— meaning the more you nurture this
connection the more you thrive.*

*Next, follow this energy up your spine and into the
crown chakra, which points up. Strands of light within
the chakra are gently and lovingly straightened and
elongated, opening your connection to Spirit. This is a
natural connection to your soul's voice, and so will
offer you much guidance if you are open to it.*

*Visualize the back of your neck lengthening as long
streams of light flow up and down the back of your
head, moving into the front of the brow chakra. As this
sixth chakra energy is cleared, you are more able to
visualize positive outcomes for the future, remembering that the future cannot be judged by the past. To do
so prevents the energy of change from flowing. As the
energy continues through the chakra and out of the
back of your head, the emotional charge of negative
ideas is released and the sixth chakra opens through
the back of your head to help you release preconceived*

*notions about yourself and
your life.*

*Follow the energy through the back of your neck into
the fifth chakra and out through the front of your
throat. Issues of worthiness and will power are held in
this chakra.*

*Move the energy into the front of the heart chakra,
softening all anxiety and worry, and allow yourself to
see a beautiful vision of your Self as Light. This is you,
having forgiven everyone and everything... including
yourself. No animosity, no regret. Feel all the systems
in your body in flow and operating optimally. And as
the energy flows through the back of the heart chakra,
your whole system feels connected and has come into
balance.*

*With each breath, take the energy out of the back of
the heart chakra, up your back and over your head,
and back into the front of the heart chakra. At the
same time, the Earth feeds her energy up the tube of
Light and throughout your field.*

The session is sealed and it is complete.

MEDITATION

*If you want to find God,
hang out in the space between your thoughts.*
—Alan Cohen

Meditation is an approach to training the mind, similar to the way
that physical exercise is an approach to training the body. It is the
practice of engaging in contemplation or inner reflection, by
concentrating on our breath, a word or an image. All the
techniques of meditation serve to open us to our fundamental
nature and the realization of ourselves as Unity consciousness.

Below are explanations of the many meditation techniques that exist, how to prepare to meditate and how to recognize if you are really in "the zone."

Popular Types of Meditation

Mental Repetition: Mental repetition means a thought is produced over and over again. It is most commonly done by the use of a mantra, which is often a one-syllable word (Om, one, peace, love, etc.) and should be done in conjunction with exhaling. A mantra can also be a short, positive phrase ("I feel good," "I am worthy of love," "My body is calm and relaxed," etc.) to reinforce positive self-esteem. This is done to clear all other thoughts from the conscious mind.

Visual concentration: Visual concentration involves focusing on or staring at an object or image. In Sanskrit, this is called *tratak*. This process involves staring at an object 3 to 5 feet away, without blinking, until it is etched on the mind's blackboard to the exclusion of all other thoughts. The suggested duration is about 60 seconds. Then close your eyes and visualize the object. Repeat if the mental image fades or vanishes.

Repeated Sounds: In some forms of meditation, sound is repeated continually to help focus the mind's attention. The Sanskrit name for this is *nadam*. Bells, a beating drum, chimes, or Gregorian chants are all examples of possible sounds to use. Sounds from nature or new age music may also be used.

Physical Repetition: This is repetitive motion such as the sensation of breathing, or some forms of rhythmic aerobic exercise (running, swimming, walking, etc.) that are believed by many to produce a meditative state ("being in the zone"), either due to the sound of breathing or the rhythmic motions of the feet or arms. Some people say their most creative thoughts come during this type of exercise.

Tactile Repetition: Holding a small object, such as a tumble stone or seashell, also brings focus to the mind. Hindu yogis use a strand of beads called a *mala*, holding it in their right hand, and rolling the beads one by one between the thumb and third finger as they meditate.

Mindfulness Meditation: This type of meditation appears to be very similar to free association, where the mind wanders aimlessly. The mind is free to accept all thoughts; no attempt is made to control the mind's content. There is one condition however: all thoughts that enter the subconscious mind must do so objectively and without judgment or emotional directive (called detached observation). In other words, do not "follow" the thoughts anywhere.

Guided Imagery: Imagery, when used to promote physical calmness, involves several components of meditation, specifically, increased concentration and expanded awareness of conscious-ness of the scene created in the mind's eye. Its greatest strength lies in the abilities to turn down the volume and intensity of information received by the five senses, and in many cases to replace negative thoughts with pleasurable ones from the depths of the imagination.

Preparation for Meditation

There are four basics steps to follow to promote a quiet, balanced mind-body. These same four components can be found in virtually every relaxation technique, from mental imagery to progressive relaxation.

- **A quiet environment:** It is best to have a quiet environment with minimal distractions.

- **A mental device:** A mental device such as any object or tool used to replace all other thoughts. It is a focal point to direct all attention. This may be breathing, the use of a mantra, or quiet music.

- **A passive attitude:** A passive attitude is a receptive attitude. It is a frame of mind in which you are open to thoughts rather than blocking them out. A passive attitude has also been interpreted as a state of physical calmness.

- **A comfortable position:** The earliest meditation advocates stated that to relax the mind, one must first relax the body. So you must first find a comfortable position.

Keys to Meditating

During meditation, some characteristics that indicate the occurrence of an altered state of consciousness have been noted. They are as follows:

- **Time Distortion:** During meditation, a distortion of time perception may occur. What may truly be an hour might feel like only twenty minutes.

- **Ineffability:** Many times, an experience will occur during mediation that you simply will not be able to put into words.

- **Present-centeredness:** The goal of meditation is to exist in the present moment—to be present and centered in the here and now.

- **Enhanced Receptivity:** The characteristic of an altered state is similar to hypnotic or subliminal suggestion; however, in meditation, the suggestions come from the inner or Higher Self.

Mind-Body Practices

■ **Self-Transcendence:** Meditation does really appear to have a mystical, spiritual quality to it. Inner peace results from the realization of unity or oneness with the Universe. When a state of super-consciousness is achieved, ego falls away, and there is the realization of a connectedness to all things.

EXPERIENCING YOUR FIVE KOSHAS

The five sheaths are not theoretical constructs. They are real parts of your being that you can actually experience.

The following exercise will help you get a fuller sense of these inner energy bodies. You can access the following online at randibotnick.com/listeninglibrary.

Sit comfortably with your head, neck, and trunk in a straight line. Close your eyes, withdrawing your awareness from the sights and sounds around you. Bring your full attention to your physical body. Be aware of your head and shoulders, chest and waist, back and abdomen, arms and legs. Turn your attention deeper inward, sensing your organs and glands. Feel the movement of the blood flowing throughout your body. Find your heartbeat. Contemplate the way all of the body's systems work in unison to create this vessel that allows you to have a physical experience on Earth. This is your annamaya kosha (physical body).

Bring your full attention to your breath. The breath (prana) is the current or presence of Source within you. Follow the breath in through your nostrils, the back of your throat and into your lungs. Slowly fill your lungs from your chest to your belly. Become aware of the energy pulsing through your body. It is making your heart beat, your lungs expand and contract, the blood course through your veins, your stomach gurgle. Feel or sense the breath moving down the spine (with the inhalation) and back up and out (with the exhalation). The force orchestrating this movement—not your physical body itself—is your pranamaya kosha (breath body).

Shift your awareness into your emotions. Reflect upon how you were feeling yesterday, or earlier today. Notice how you are feeling now, in this moment. Remember that the emotions communicate to us important information, both positive and negative, about our needs and boundaries. This is your manomaya kosha (emotional body).

Lift your awareness higher inside your skull by rolling your eyes up inside your lids. Sense the part of your awareness that consciously made the decision to participate in this exercise. It recognizes the value of expanding your self-awareness and compels you to find positive tools for your self-improvement and spiritual education. At the same time, recognize the stillness that exists in the background. The stillness is the connection to the "Great Mind," the source of all wisdom. This is your vijnanamaya kosha (intellect body).

Center your awareness in your heart. Relax deeply; keep breathing smoothly and evenly. Now, taking as much time as you need, visualize an idyllic field of green grass. Emanating up out of the Earth is a beautiful fountain of water. As you watch the water surge and dance, the fountain begins to grow in size, radiating a sense of joy, love and peace. Allow yourself to settle into a state of complete tranquility... a space of perfect contentment, perfect attunement, and abiding stillness. There is no sense of lack, or fear, or desire. You are a separate identity immersed within the Unity of All That Is. This is your anandamaya kosha (bliss body).

Now simply be aware of your own awareness—the pure consciousness that is having this experience, that lies beyond this experience. It is your true inner Self, your immortal being. Rest in your own being for as long as you can hold your attention there.

Return your attention to your breath. Breathe slowly, smoothly, and evenly. Gently open your eyes. Take a moment to relax and absorb this experience before you get up.

Mind-Body Practices

GROUNDING EXERCISE

This exercise helps us create a conscious connection between our bodies, the Earth and Spirit. From this place of connection we can more easily move about our lives with ease and grace.

Those of us who are highly sensitive can often feel ungrounded. This may be caused by any kind of stress— environmental, physical, emotional or mental. Some symptoms of being ungrounded include feeling spacey, forgetting things, losing things, clumsiness, and anxiety.

You may choose to record this visualization for ease of practice or access the following online at randibotnick.com/ listeninglibrary.

Sit in a chair or on the couch with your feet flat on the floor, or sit in a comfortable cross-legged position. Close your eyes and begin to relax and center yourself by following your breath.

When your mind has quieted down, begin to visualize roots growing from the bottom of your feet (if you are seated in a chair) or from the backs of your legs (if you are seated cross-legged). Watch as the roots slowly grow down into the Earth. Watch as the roots become longer and longer, gradually moving towards the Earth's core. When the roots reach the core, feel the pulse of the Earth's energy and slowly begin to draw that energy up through the roots into your body.

Feel the Earth energy pulsing through your body, as it moves up your legs, into your trunk, and begins to spread throughout your chakras and into all of your organs and into your arms. Sit for a few moments connecting with this energy.

Imagine that your body is made up of a grid of Light... and that grid is connected to an even greater grid that is connected to the Earth and all her inhabitants. Follow the lines of your grid to the core—or the heart—of the Earth. The pulse of her heartbeat is pure and constant. Allow the pulse of the planet to reverberate throughout your energy field.

Now, visualize strands of silver and gold reaching out from the crown of your head towards the sky. Watch as these cords slowly begin to climb towards Source Creator. As these silver and gold cords connect with the All, allow yourself to fill with the high vibration of this Universal energy. Allow this energy to begin to travel through the cords, moving slowly down towards your body.

Feel the Universal energy entering through the crown of your head. Visualize this energy moving down through your body and pulsating out through your chakras, your arms, your internal organs, and down your legs.

Now allow the Earth energy and the Universal energy to merge. Feel your own energy as both of these fill you.

Sit for as long as you would like. When you are ready, slowly open your eyes.

TRANSMUTING NEGATIVE THOUGHTS

We all suffer from negative thoughts at times. Turning inward and creating a stronger, more positive frame of mind - and even a wonderful fantasy of the future - is the best remedy to regain balance.

Enlarging positive representations of who you really are and how you fit into the world, and bringing these closer into your field of inner vision, while, quite literally, making smaller the representations of those beliefs that no longer serve you, is one powerful, yet easy, exercise. Your subconscious mind has no way to know the difference between what is true reality and what is imagination, so it can do nothing but believe the new, positive visions, just as it has believed negative thoughts in the past.

Mind-Body Practices

Here are three more quick and easy ways to relieve yourself of negative thoughts and boost your vibration.

- **Visualize a Good Vibration**
  Practice visually changing the vibration of any negative thoughtform or emotion. Use visualization to "paint" the uncomfortable pocket of energy with a bright, vibrant color that feels good. Imagine a can of spray paint or a roller, and cover the negative thoughtform or emotion with the beautiful color.

- **Overwrite Negative Feelings**
  Quiet your mind.

  Locate the uncomfortable energy. Where do you feel it in or on your body?

  Find a positive and powerful image or memory of yourself, one in which you are in your mastery. Notice how that feels.

  Place the positive image on top of the negative feeling. Wait as the negative feeling dissipates.

- **Boost Your Energy Field**
  Do this to quickly raise your vibration:

  Imagine that your energy field is a balloon and, using your breath, expand your field.

  Ask to connect to all the beings and energies that are here to love and support you. (Trust me—there is a multitude!) Spend a few minutes basking in the energies of Love.

10. Emotional Release Processes

What if the genesis of disease happened because
of emotions that were unrecognized, unacknowledged
and unexpressed?

A t the core of holistic healing is the structured release of
pent-up emotions. When ignored, these emotions may
create anxiety, panic attacks, prolonged depression, or a
multitude of stress-related ailments.

While whatever feelings arise must be accepted and acknowl-
edged, we run the risk of getting stuck in the "story" of our
wounding. For decades it was helpful to "process" our feelings
and uncover the core wound or trauma. In this day and age, as the
veil thins and we have more access to the Light that is our Divine
Selves, it has become less necessary to spend years processing
painful feelings and, instead, find ways to release them.

> *Years ago I was on the verge of going into business*
> *with a partner. We had been planning this for months,*
> *talking at length about where we would practice, what*
> *it would look like, how we would share responsibilities.*
> *On the eve of signing the contract, however, my*
> *partner pulled out. But not only did he pull out, he*
> *signed on with two other people instead. I was*
> *devastated.*
>
> *All of my visions of my future were shattered, my*
> *expectations crushed. Psychologically I receded into my*
> *childhood wounds of not being accepted, not fitting in,*
> *and not being loved. Spiritually, I was reliving past*
> *lifetimes of similar betrayal by the same souls.*
> *Mentally, I understood this was the best possible*
> *outcome, but emotionally I was overwhelmed with*
> *anger that I could not seem to release.*

133

Foundations of Energy Healing

For months I struggled, vacillating between expressing my rage and then suppressing it and pretending I was fine. Finally, a good friend of mine advised me to allow myself to just Be... to feel my feelings without judgment as they arose, and likewise, witness them release as they settled down. This mindfulness practice was the beginning of my healing. I let go of the "story" of my pain and my need to understand it and process it over and over again. Instead, as I stayed focused on the present, I was able to find ways to quiet my mind and create more positive thoughts. I was ultimately able to devise a new future plan, one in which I could appreciate my newfound freedom.

There is a great deal of impelling information on forgiveness, but I believe that forgiveness comes after allowing ourselves to accept our emotional responses, no matter how dark. We must have time to grieve or rage or feel *everything* first.

Ultimately, understand that, even while feeling it all, we are not the feelings; we are merely having the feelings. ("I am angry" is different from "I feel angry.") Therefore, developing a consistent practice of meditation, visualization and emotional release techniques leads to more permanent inner quiet, contentment and optimism.

Following are various practices designed to calm the mind by creating new, more positive thoughts.

VOW RELEASE[1]

Throughout our many lifetimes, we have taken numerous vows of control. Most of the time, a person had an intense karmic experience, died, hit the lower astral plane and vowed, "I'm never going to do that again!"

Vows can also be taken during this lifetime and previous lifetimes, as well as in the astral plane. For example, a scorned lover might declare, "I will never love again!" or "I will always wait for him." Think of all the times you have said, "I will never

134

…. again" or "I will always…." Situations or experiences that we vowed we would never experience again were essentially vows to not follow Spirit.

You can begin to identify vows by noticing repetitive patterns in your, or a client's, life. Perhaps someone who cannot seem to eke out a living took a vow of poverty at some point. A person who has recurrent sexual dysfunction may have taken a vow of chastity. Or someone who is perpetually abused by her bosses may have taken a vow of subservience.

Once identified, it is best to consciously rescind the vows. Follow the method below to do so.

State:

I rescind any and all vows, contracts, agreements, or oaths I have taken, anyone in this body has taken and anyone within my genetic lineage has taken pertaining to

State vows here: (See "Suggested Vows," below, or include your own.) …………………………………..

I now declare these vows, contracts, agreements, or oaths, null and void in this incarnation and all incarnations across all space and all time, all parallel realities, all parallel universes, all alternate realities, all alternate universes, all planetary systems, all source systems, all dimensions and the Void.
Spirit, please release all structures, devices, entities, orientations, beliefs, behaviors, cellular memory, crystalline thought forms, closed systems, pictures of reality, telepathic images, emotions, energetics, or effects associated with these vows, contracts, agree-ments, or oaths NOW!

And so it is!

Suggested Vows:

- Going to sleep and forgetting who I AM
- Participating with limitation

- Making limitation real
- Not following Spirit
- Not trusting the movement of Spirit
- Denying karmic interaction
- Not recognizing karmic monads
- Using karma for intensity
- Using polarity to search for oneness
- Resisting Divinity, Infinity, and Ecstasy
- Upholding the original Prime Directive of Survival: procreation, territoriality and defense against the enemy
- Holding childhood imprinting in place
- Resentment, anger, lack of forgiveness, pity, martyrdom, manipulation, coercion, collusion, and conditionality
- Denying the mastery of myself or others
- Denying the sovereignty of myself or others
- Not recognizing or using divine law and principle
- Keeping chakras and lower bodies separated
- Ignoring a given chakra or body
- Resisting vertical, transpersonal positioning
- Resisting communion with Spirit
- Resisting full embodiment of Spirit

SUPERCONSCIOUS TECHNIQUE[2]

After rescinding vows, use this technique to institute new, conscious intentions. List as many as you would like. By Universal Law, no higher-dimensional being can intercede or assist you unless you request it. Develop the habit of asking for assistance, information and guidance. Let your guides know that you are ready for positive change!

State:

Superconscious, by the Force of Grace, will you manifest the essence of the performance and effect, and embodiment of the highest possibilities of

State intentions here: (See "Suggested Intentions" below, or include your own.) ....

So that the power of that can be manifest fully in my experience. And so it is! NOW!

Suggested Intentions:

- Taking care of myself
- Forming friendships easily
- Standing in my power
- Speaking my truth
- Being allowed to have what I want
- Deserving the best
- Being deserving of and receptive to kindness
- Being whole and complete within myself
- Being loved and appreciated by others
- Inviting and allowing good to come into my life
- Other people valuing and honoring my worth
- Loving myself
- Deserving to be happy
- Believing in myself
- Recognizing my successes
- Knowing God
- Participating in life

- Knowing I AM loved
- Trusting myself fully
- Knowing I AM whole and healed
- Seeing the world through a mature lens
- Accepting and loving myself just as I AM
- Owning and standing in my power
- Knowing who I AM at all levels
- Fully integrating who I AM upper-dimensionally
- Moving forward with confidence and joy
- Being open to all the abundance of the universe
- Believing in myself
- Speaking my truth with certainty
- Being strong and healthy

Note: When you feel like you are manifesting what you don't want, say:

"Superconscious—manifested illusion—course correct now!"

"Powerful You" Visualization

This technique is helpful for increasing self-esteem and offering a different possibility for a stressful situation. You can access the following online at randibotnick.com/listeninglibrary for yourself, or use the script below for your clients. If doing this for yourself, record your answers so you can review them later.

First, have your client close her eyes, and explain that you are going to guide her through a visualization that asks her to use her imagination. While you are guiding her, ask her to hold her eyes in different positions through this visualization. In the directions below, the eye positions will be described by combination of letters, using the following: "**D**" = "down," "**U**" = "up," "**L**" =

"left," "**R**" = "right," "**C**" = "center." Visualizing images while holding the eyes in different positions re-patterns the brain. Recite the following:

D-R:

> *Begin to imagine yourself at your most powerful. As much as possible, imagine that part of yourself that holds your highest knowledge, the highest part of your being. There is no right answer. You might see a cartoon character, a super hero, or just you at your best. Observe what comes to you.*

D-C:

> *Now, take whatever feeling, sense or glimpse you've gotten of this, and actually see yourself with this characteristic within you. Either focus on your body or examine yourself as if you were looking in a mirror, but however you choose, look at your physical structure and look at the energy that surrounds you. How do you look as you observe yourself? Observe what you are experiencing.*

D-L:

> *Allow yourself to really get a feeling of what this is like in a physical form. Feel your power in your body. Observe what this feels like.*

U-R:

> *Now allow this powerful self to take some kind of action, to do something. This may be a small gesture or a grand movement. What do you do?*

U-C:

> *What are the results of the action you have taken? Observe the results you have gotten.*

U-L:

> *Now just allow yourself to be alone as this Powerful You, to be alone in a space of your own. Become even more aware of your own knowing, and your own loving, with no one else around. Observe what this feels like.*

U-C:

> *Now allow yourself, as this Powerful You, to be in the presence of Higher Beings, others that are all-knowing,*

and that are all love. Allow as many of them as you like to be there with you. Become aware of what it is like for you there, and what it is like for them to be in your presence and in your energy.

(Long pause.)

Now allow this combination of all the energy that is now present to become aware of an even greater and broader sense of what is all-knowing and all-loving. Allow all those present to become aware of the Universal Love, of what might be referred to as God, or whatever higher power you believe in. Allow this energy of the entire universe that is loving and positive to be with you

D-C:

Get a good grasp of what this experience is like, and bring this experience down into your physical body, in this time and place. Own this experience; make it a part of you. Move this feeling into any part of you that feels tense or tight. Fill those areas with this loving energy.

"HIGHER SELF" IMAGERY

This technique is helpful for relieving depression and remembering that we are always much more than our physical selves. You can access the following online at randibotnick.com/listeninglibrary to use for yourself, or the read script below for your clients. If doing this for yourself, record your answers so you can review them later.

First, have your client close her eyes, and explain that you are going to guide her through a visualization that asks her to use her imagination. While you are guiding her, ask her to hold her eyes in different positions through this visualization. In the directions below, the eye positions will be described by combination of letters, using the following: "**D**" = "down," "**U**" = "up," "**L**" =

"left," "**R**" = "right," "**C**" = "center," "**E**" = "ear." Visualize the following:

D-R:

> *Observe your Higher Self in whatever form that takes for you. Be aware of the images and feelings that come to you as your Higher Self. Observe what comes to you.*

D-C:

> *What does your Higher Self feel like? Observe what feeling comes to you.*

D-L:

> *Allow your Higher Self to do something... to go into action. This may be a small gesture or a grand movement. What action does your Higher Self take?*

U-R:

> *What sound is associated with your Higher Self?*

U-C:

> *Bring intellect and intelligence into this experience of your Higher Self. How does your Higher Self use your intelligence? What does it use your intelligence for?*

U-L:

> *What smell, fragrance or scent is associated with your Higher Self?*

R-E:

> *Bring intuition into this experience of your Higher Self. How does your higher self use your intuition? What does it use your intuition for?*

L-E:

> *Bring logic into this experience of your Higher Self. How does your Higher Self use logic? What does it use logic for?*

U-C:

Now combine the feeling with sound, smell, intellect, knowing and logic. Allow all of these attributes to join together at once in your experience. What is this like for your Higher Self?

Bring into your experience the highest energy forms you can conceive and allow them to interact with your Higher Self. What is your Higher Self's experience of this interaction? How do the higher energy beings feel about you?

D-C:

Now grasping the wholeness of that experience of your complete Higher Self in interaction, bring that Self down into your physical body at this time and place. Examine your physical body to see if there is any tension, pain or stress anywhere in it. If there is, allow the Higher Self to go to the place or part and just rest and inhabit that area. Fill that area with the experience of your Higher Self. Allow your Higher Self to fill your physical body completely. Experience that Self within your physical body.

U-C:

Bring the wholeness of your Higher Self experience as you turn your eyes up. What color is associated with your Higher Self?

D-C:

Now allow this color to join the experience of your Higher Self, bring this whole experience down into your physical body, and allow the Higher Self's color to spread throughout your whole body, filling it completely.

Then, when you are ready, gently open your eyes and return to this time and place.

Include the information gleaned from this visualization in your daily life to remind you of your connection to your Higher Self. For example:

- Return to the sensation of the wholeness of this experience;

Emotional Release Processes

- Visualize the color flowing through your body before going to sleep at night or before getting out of bed in the morning; or

- Re-invoke the color and sound that best describe your Higher Self.

PROGRESSIVE RELAXATION

This is a process you can do for yourself or your client to help facilitate the relaxation response. Many people have been living in the stress response for so long that they have forgotten what it feels like to be relaxed. This helps the mind and body remember how it feels to be calm so the body can move out of the stress response loop. I recommend recording this so you can listen to it with your eyes closed or use my recording online at randibotnick.com/listeninglibrary.

Begin by finding a comfortable place to lie down with your eyes closed. Adjust yourself anyway you need to feel completely comfortable and supported.

(Pause.)

Begin by taking three very deep, full breaths.

(Pause for the three breaths.)

Follow the movement of your breath as your body expands on the inhalations...and contracts and relaxes on the exhalations.... Allow your breath to slow down so that the exhalations are longer than the inhalations.

(Pause.)

Withdraw yourself from your environment... Withdraw yourself from your surroundings... Withdraw yourself from all sounds around you, except for the sound of my voice. And the sound of my voice will follow you wherever you go. And if your mind begins to wander, then that's OK. It just means you're relaxing and feeling very languid. In fact, your conscious mind may not hear everything that I say... and that's OK because your subconscious mind is open and receptive to all of my suggestions here.

So bring your attention to your feet and toes. There's an energy moving into the soles of your feet, and that energy is relaxing all the muscles in your feet and toes. Feel the muscles relax now....

That energy is moving up into your calves, and as it moves, both of your calf muscles become quite loose and relaxed. Feel your calf muscles relax now.... The energy is moving now into your thigh muscles, causing them to simply let go and become loose.... Now that relaxing energy is moving into your hips and groin, and the muscles there also unwind and become loose and relaxed.... And that same soothing, relaxing energy flows into your buttocks, and those muscles also relax....

Feel the energy moving now, and it's moving into your abdominal muscles, waist, and the small of your back. As it does, all the muscles there are bathed in relaxing energy, which causes them to unwind like a rubber band letting go.

(Pause.)

Now this soothing, relaxing energy is flowing up into your chest and upper back, causing the muscles there to become loose and limp and relaxed.... The energy is moving into your shoulders now, and as your muscles relax, you can feel your shoulders sink down.... Follow the energy down your arms, hands, and fingers, relaxing all of those muscles. You may feel warmth in the palms of your hands; you may even feel some tingling in your fingertips as the energy reaches them.

(Pause.)

That same relaxing energy is now moving into your neck, and if you are holding any tension there, it simply dissipates, allowing the neck muscles to become loose and free.... The energy is now moving into your head, causing the muscles on your scalp and around your ears to unwind and it may even feel like your scalp is sliding down.... Feel the energy flowing around your face, and as it moves, all the tiny muscles around your eyes, nose, and mouth let go.... And it flows into the cheeks and jaw.... lips and tongue.

(Pause.)

Your entire body is now totally relaxed, your entire body is now totally relaxed, your entire body is now totally relaxed. You are feeling drowsy, and comfortable, and secure. That energy is still in you and is now flowing out of the top of your head and is moving down towards your feet. As it reaches your feet, your entire body is now enveloped in a warm cocoon of energy that protects you from any negative influences.

Enjoy this experience of relaxation: so quiet, so peaceful.

Pause for up to 15 minutes. (Our recording pauses for 10 minutes.)

Slowly begin coming back now, bringing your awareness back to your surroundings. As you awaken, be aware of how nice it feels to be this relaxed, this peaceful. These feelings of peace and calm and relaxation will remain with you all day and into the evening. These feelings are yours.
Become aware of yourself here, in this place, at this time.... Take a deep full breath.... Wiggle your fingers and toes.... And gently, when you are ready, slowly open your eyes, coming back fully awake, aware and alert, but remaining peaceful and calm for the rest of the day and into the evening.

INNER CHILD

As children, when we experience a trauma, or anything that feels traumatic, and we do not have help with processing, understanding or discharging the resulting feelings, a part of our ego becomes frozen in that time. Psychologically, the subconscious mind registers a danger and the reaction to it. The subconscious mind then continues to replay the same scenario over and over again anytime we have an experience that reminds of us the initial trauma (often called an imprint). Sometimes this is interpreted as the inner child getting "frozen" at that maturity level and no longer advancing.

Inner Child work is a way to safely tap into the initial imprint and heal the part that has stayed frozen in that experience. To access your subconscious mind, you must be in an altered state. So begin by practicing the Progressive Relaxation. Alternately, close your eyes and breathe evenly and deeply for five minutes to quiet your mind.

Notice how you feel. What is the predominant feeling that arises? To begin to name the feeling, use this list:

- *Scared*
- *Sad*
- *Mad*
- *Guilty*
- *Hurt*
- *Lonely*
- *Confused*

Notice where this feeling sits in your body.

Describe this feeling as a color, shape or image (purple, a cloud, a snarling dog, etc.).

Describe this feeling as a sensation (knotted, tight, congested, swirling, etc.)

How old were you when you felt this feeling for the very first time?

Visualize yourself at that age.

If that child were your son/daughter, would you love him/her? If so, tell the child that you love him/her, and why. State, "I love you because...."

Let the child recount any story about the feelings. What happened to cause it? Where were you? Who else was there? Allow the child to share the story and the resulting feelings with total freedom.

(Note: Do not judge anything the child feels or says. Do not tell the child to stop feeling that way. Do not tell the child to go away.)

Tell the child two things: "You survived it and it is over. I know you survived it, because I am you, all grown up." And "It's not your fault."

Ask the child, "What do you need from me now to feel better?" Once you have the answer, notice what it would feel like to receive that. And notice how your body feels. For example, your child may want a hug or to go to a playground. Offer her that experience in your imagination.

Ask the child again, "What else do you need from me?" Keep asking and giving the child what he/she needs until the child feels complete.

Now create a safe place for the child. This may be a favorite place outside, like a playground, or it may be a familiar place inside, like the kitchen in Grandmother's house. Wherever it is, bring the child there. Be detailed: What does it look like? What does it feel like? What smells are there? What do you hear around you?

Allow the child to get comfortable there, to do something fun or find a safe place to rest before opening your eyes and returning to a fully awake state.

147

Foundations of Energy Healing

INTENTIONS AND AFFIRMATIONS

Affirmations allow us to paint a picture of our hopes and dreams… to set our intentions for how we want to create our perceptions and realities. Intentions should be specific, and stated positively in the present tense and the first person ("I" statements). Refrain from saying anything like, "I am not stressed." Instead, find the positive way to claim that, such as, "I am calm and centered," or "I sleep deeply every night."

I recommend that you record this and listen to it every day. Play it in your car or in the background while you are working around the house, or just before bed. Each time you listen to your intentions, your energy expands and rises, opening the doors for all good things to enter (as is in alignment with your highest good).

Here is an example of a set of intentions and affirmations. Use any statements that you feel fit for you. Make it as long as you like, including all aspects of your life that you want addressed. And then change (and re-record) them as you need.

I am peaceful and content in my life. My mind is clear and calm and open to see all of the possibilities in my life. I keep my eye on the prize, my biggest goals, and I aim for those goals.

Life is really good. I enjoy my days and I am happy to be alive. My days are filled with the perfect work/play balance. I am stimulated in my business, and calm and happy in my personal life. I feel more confident than ever before, and that shows in the way I communicate with ease and presence in conversation, at home and at work.

All of my decision-making comes from a grounded, calm place. Whether I am talking to a friend, talking about important issues with my spouse, speaking to my family, making business decisions, managing the household, or managing my money, I am centered and receptive to my intuition and my knowing.

I enter a room with an expanded energy field and my head up, and when I speak, I look people in the eye. I have a newfound trust in the world. I feel strong within myself. Because I now know who I am, I come across in conversations as holding my power. I am confident, I know who I am and what I have to offer. My friends and family see this about me, and marvel at how much I've changed. I am proud of myself.

I now have more than enough money to buy whatever I need and want, and I am putting 10% of my income into savings. I now have enough money to support my family and myself. I can afford to buy my own house, to treat myself to vacations, to socialize, and to eat dinners out with friends. I am free to have fun every week. I am happy knowing that I am independent and secure.

I feel fulfilled as I go to work each day, knowing I am needed. I feel smart as I take on new and old tasks with ease. I allow all of my talents to shine through. I am great with people. I am patient. I am compassionate. I choose to help out in any way that I can.

I spend my days calm and relaxed. I have lots of energy to do all the things I need and want to do. I sleep very well at night, leaving the day behind, and feel rested and energized when I wake up in the morning. This happens too, because my home is peaceful, and my mind reflects that. I can be myself at home, I can relax and take care of myself in my own unique ways. I belong here, and I know it's okay to be myself in whatever way that shows up each day. I have the perfect balance between self-care and care of others.

I am more able to trust myself and stand in my power in all my relationships at home. I am connected to my children and responsive and receptive to their needs. I am a compassionate and loving parent. My relationships with my family members are easy and we have fun with each other.

I am in a loving, caring and supportive relationship. My partner and I are good friends and communicate with ease. We are open to hearing each other's points of view and coming to the best decisions for the relationship. Our life is a collaboration, and we are a team. We are passionate with each other mentally and physically. There is a true respect between us and we consider ourselves equals.

ENDNOTES: CHAPTER 10

1. Published with permission from JJ Wilson and Alchemical Mage Tools & Techniques. www.alchemicalmage.com/tools/index.htm.

2. Printed with permission from Alchemical Mage, based on tools from E.T. Earth Mission. www.alchemicalmage.com/tools/index.htm.

11. Energy Release Processes

*What if subtle energy disturbances were
at the root of the suffering we experience?*

This section contains invocations and prayers that call on various teams of angels, archangels and elohim to clear energies in and around your body and personal spaces. Specifically, these different invocations affect your energy bodies, relationships and personal spaces, keeping them clean and clear of negative patterns and imprints.

These are invaluable for your own daily personal use, assuring more ease in your life, physically, mentally and emotionally. Introduce them to your clients as well for added value in their sessions.

SWEEPING THE ENERGY FIELD

This technique is very simple, yet extremely effective at clearing the entire body of congested energy. As the energy is moved and cleared, your client will feel calmer, quieter and more relaxed. Sweeping the field improves both physical and etheric energy flow, and you will likely observe changes in your client's breath, skin color and pulse rate.

Bring your hands about 3 or 4 inches above the body and move your hands slightly until you feel the etheric field. Wherever you feel a disturbance, a block or a condensation of energy, work this area by moving the hands in any direction following the energy flow. You may use the palms of your hand, your fingers, or your etheric fingers (imagining extending the energy of your fingers deep into the energy body).

Brush the energy with your palms, or comb and untangle it with your fingers. Open and release any pockets of condensed energy with the goal of making the field balanced and uniform.

Imagine your hands as magnets, and the debris in the energy field like iron filings that are attracted to the magnet and stick to it.

Each stroke may feel different as new layers are reached. Move your hands through the etheric body, the mental body, the emotional body and the spiritual body.

Trust the energy as a guide. Follow it by moving your hands in the client's field for as long as necessary (even the whole session!) until the field feels completely clear and smooth.

Trauma Energy Release

As mentioned in Chapter 7, Clearing Trauma, our etheric bodies have accumulated trauma through our many lifetimes, as well as through our genes. This often feels like blockages or condensation in the energy body. The energy of these traumas may show up as physical pain and illness, emotional fears or negative self-talk. During a session, your client may call your attention to pain in the body, or your guides may direct you to an area that needs to be cleared.

Trauma from past lives most often sits in the part of the body that received a physical wound. For instance,

I was working on a client who wanted to be as clear as possible as she moved into a new line of work. I was guided to work on what psychically looked like a black scar across the back of her neck, even though she had no pain there. I saw that this wound in her neck was related to a past life scenario in which she was beheaded. In that lifetime she was a well-to-do young

*woman, living in a castle. I distinctly saw her beautiful
light-green silk gown.*

*She was spinning silk to weave with, and she made such
beautiful silk that she was thought to have magical
powers. This terrified the others in the castle, and so
she was put to death.*

*Although the trauma had not physically manifested as
pain or any other kind of ailment in her current
lifetime, I was given the information that the fear and
anger that situation caused might infiltrate in this next
phase of her life. There was a potential that she would
hold herself back from the fear of being killed for her
gifts.*

How To Release Trauma Energy

You will be guided as to where this energy is located in the body.
Then pull the energy out like you would gather and pull taffy. You
can either work directly in your client's etheric field, or visualize
your client's body as if it were in front of you and work on it
holographically. Take your time and work slowly. Trauma energy
may sit deep inside the body, or far in the energy field. It may
have roots or tendrils that wrap around body parts. Be careful to
get it all. Muscle test—or ask your guides in any way that is best
for you—if it is all clear.

Once it is removed, the healing team will fill that area with
healing light. They may ask you to place your hands on or over
the area, move your hands in specific patterns, or they may do all
that is needed themselves.

Remember, it's all about the intention you have. When you
remain clear, the operation is effective.

Foundations of Energy Healing

CUTTING CORDS AND RELEASING KARMIC TIES

Another important technique is cutting cords that negatively bind people to current or previous relationships and prevent them from being present with, or completing, those relationships in the highest of ways. Some of the emotions and interactions that create cords include:

- Anger
- Abuse
- Co-dependence
- Fear
- Guilt
- Neediness
- Unrequited love
- Vows and promises

These cords, and the resulting psychic attachments and karmic ties, exist across and beyond lifetimes. Therefore, leaving the cords intact often results in repeating similar patterns...a karmic loop, so to speak.

Cutting these cords does not necessarily mean that we are severing our relationships. It may mean that these relationships will evolve into unconditionally loving and accepting ones, from a place of wholeness and free will.

State:

I release my needs to project fear and keep myself from the Love that I AM. I release my needs to please. I release my addictions. I release my fears. And in so doing, I release the ties that bind.

I ask for the gentle release of all that I am holding onto between me and .... not of

154

God's desire, in this incarnation and all incarnations across all space and all time, all parallel realities, all parallel universes, all alternate realities, all alternate universes, all planetary systems, all source systems, all dimensions and the Void.

Pause until the release feels complete.

Spirit, please release all structures, devices, entities, orientations, beliefs, behaviors, cellular memories, crystalline thought forms, closed systems, pictures of reality, telepathic images, emotions, energetics, or effects associated with these cords.

When that feels complete, say "Thank you."

TRIPLE GRIDS[1]

The Triple Grid technique is for keeping areas like your home, workplace or car energetically clean. Ask each specific group of angels to set up its level of the grid, designating the geometric shape, size and location. Spherical grids are the most stable and easy to maintain, so it is suggested that you work with this geometry for most everyday applications (such as around your home, car or workplace). You will want to renew the grid weekly or whenever you notice the energy getting out of sorts.

The grid can also be programmed into a quartz crystal. This can be done by holding the crystal (preferably a sphere) and setting your intent to program the grid into the crystal while saying the Triple Grid technique. The grid is maintained by the Deva of the crystal. Just keeping the crystal in your home, car, office, or other location, will perpetuate the energies of the grid.

Devas are the consciousness of the crystals; the spirits, the minds and souls of the stones. They are individual spiritual, mental, and emotional aspects of each crystal or stone. They are the collective mind of each kind of stone. Crystal Devas are the over-lighting essence and unified consciousness of all crystals and stones and all that pertains or relates to stones. Crystal Devas are a manifestation of the undifferentiated creative source, law, rhythm, power, of the Universe. They are the aware, conscious energy of the crystals manifesting in a way that enables us to better communicate or understand (or at least conceive of) what it is they are and how to work with them and the physical form of the rocks crystals and minerals.[2]

Following are four Grid Techniques: the Triple Grid and the Quad Grid Version are for your spaces. The Triple Grid: Individual Field Version and the Quad Grid: Individual Field Version are for your body. Use the one that best suits your needs at any time.

The suggestions of what energies and issues to be released and those to be infused are merely suggestions. Use those along with anything else that comes to mind for you.

The Triple Grid

The following example uses "my house," but you can substitute that with the car, office, school, or other location.
State:

Legions of Michael: grid level one, spherical, my house. Destroyer Force Angels: grid level two, spherical, my house. Circle Security: grid level three, spherical, my house.

Destroyer Force Angels: please spin your grid, spinning out astral entities, adverse electromagnetic frequencies, fear, disharmony, anger, adverse astrological influences, expectation, frustration, viruses, fungi, bacteria, worry, astral distortions, miscommunication, sadness, enemy patterning, scarcity, loneliness, karmic monads, and anything that distorts the spiritual signature or clear communication with Spirit. Spin out anything that hasn't been mentioned in this or any other language, but which you know needs to leave the space at this time."

(These are just a few suggestions. Fill in whatever is needed according to your situation).

When the clearing feels complete, continue with, *"Reverse spin, same stuff."* When that clearing feels complete, end with, *"Stop spin. Thank you."*

Legions of Michael: please infuse your grid with the energies of Grace, Purity, Faith, Hope, Peace, Liberty, Harmony, Love, Mercy, Alpha/Omega, Rapture and Victory Elohim. Infuse with love, intimacy, the Unified Chakra, centeredness, clarity, full connection with Spirit, tolerance, clear communication, health, wealth, following Spirit without hesitation, mastery, sovereignty, living Heaven, and anything else that hasn't been mentioned in this or any other language, but which you know needs to be in the space at this time.

Please seal your grid. Thank you.

(Again these are mere suggestions. Fill in whatever you need, according to your situation.)

Circle Security: Realign your grid to harmonize with upper-dimensional gridworks. Release all distortions and parasites on the grids. Infuse frequencies for clearer communication with Spirit.

Please seal your grid. Thank you.

NOTE: The Triple Grid can be done around a location without you being physically there. Try doing it around the mall, the courthouse, the grocery store or the post office, before you get there. Remember that this technique cannot be used to manipulate others; it just makes particular energies more or less easily available. This is a very versatile technique. We have given you the everyday applications. The spherical geometry is very stable and easy to maintain. Live in it all the time and it will be easier to live Heaven on Earth.

Foundations of Energy Healing

Quad Grid Version

This is an expansion of the Triple Grid, where you request assistance for dealing with the electromagnetic anomalies and surges that are currently very active on the planet. As the planet approaches Zero Point magnetics, electromagnetic surges are very common. This addition to the Triple Grid will help you keep your fields healthy through the planetary shifts.

The Ze'Or Continuum is a group of beings that originate from another universe. They are pure-energy beings, and they are the sentient embodiment of physical forces, such as gravity, electricity, magnetics, thermals, and so on. They have come to assist Earth and her inhabitants through the electromagnetic shifts we are experiencing preparatory to Zero Point. They are always available to assist upon request.

Request the Triple Grid as normal, adding a line for the Ze'Or Continuum in the beginning:

> *Legions of Michael: grid level one, spherical, my house. Destroyer Force Angels: grid level two, spherical, my house. Ze'Or Continuum: grid level three, spherical, my house. Circle Security: grid level four, spherical, my house. "*

> *Destroyer Force Angels: please spin your grid, spinning out astral entities, adverse electromagnetic frequencies, fear, disharmony, anger, adverse astrological influences, expectation, frustration, viruses, fungi, bacteria, worry, astral distortions, miscommunication, sadness, enemy patterning, scarcity, loneliness, karmic monads, and anything that distorts the spiritual signature or clear communication with Spirit. Spin out anything that hasn't been mentioned in this or any other language, but which you know needs to leave the space at this time. "*

(These are just a few suggestions. Fill in whatever is needed according to your situation).

Energy Release Processes

When the clearing feels complete, continue with, "*Reverse spin, same stuff.*" When that clearing feels complete, end with, "*Stop spin. Thank you.*"

Legions of Michael: please infuse your grid with the energies of Grace, Purity, Faith, Hope, Peace, Liberty, Harmony, Love, Mercy, Alpha/Omega, Rapture and Victory Elohim. Infuse with love, intimacy, the Unified Chakra, centeredness, clarity, full connection with Spirit, tolerance, clear communication, health, wealth, following Spirit without hesitation, mastery, sovereignty, living Heaven, and anything else that hasn't been mentioned in this or any other language, but which you know needs to be in the space at this time.

Please seal your grid. Thank you.

(Again these are mere suggestions. Fill in whatever you need, according to your situation.)

Ze'Or Continuum: please set your grid for harmonization and optimization of electrical, magnetic, and gravitational frequencies. Please ensure that my fields remain harmonized with all of the electronic and mechanical devices in my space, and that I and the devices in my space remain harmonized in frequency with any electromagnetic surges, ley-line activity, Schumann Resonance, and any other electro-magneto-gravitational events and conditions occurring in this area. Thank you.

Circle Security: realign your grid to harmonize with upper-dimensional gridworks. Release all distortions and parasites on the grids. Infuse frequencies for clearer communication with Spirit.

Please seal your grid. Thank you.

For a quick EMF adjustment, such as when you are working near computers and other electronic devices (including the chips in your vehicles, pagers, cellular phones, cordless phones, etc.), state:
Ze'Or Continuum, please assist: please harmonize the frequencies of all electronic devices in my space to this field.

159

Foundations of Energy Healing

Triple Grid: Individual Field Version

Some people have felt that the Triple Grid should NOT be used around your own fields, as the speed with which the Destroyer Forces spin might cause your own fields to fray. If the version using the Destroyer Force Angels feels too intense, use one of the next two techniques to grid your own fields.

State:

> *Legions of Michael: grid level one, spherical, my fields.*
> *Grace Elohim: grid level two, spherical, my fields.*
> *Circle Security: grid level three, spherical, my fields.*
>
> *Grace Elohim: please fill your grid with your energies, releasing astral entities, adverse electromagnetic frequencies, fear, disharmony, anger, adverse astrological influences, expectation, frustration, viruses, fungi, bacteria, worry, astral distortions, miscommunication, sadness, enemy patterning, scarcity, loneliness, karmic monads, and anything that distorts the spiritual signature or clear communication with Spirit. Release anything that hasn't been mentioned in this or any other language, but which you know needs to leave my fields at this time.*

(These are just a few suggestions. Fill in whatever is needed according to your situation.)

> *Then, "Spirit: I ask you to release all energies, entities, thought forms, emotions, cellular memories, orientations, pictures of reality, devices, intrusions and effects in my body and fields that are not of my core Divine essence, NOW!*

When the clearing feels complete, continue with, *"Reverse spin, same stuff."* When that clearing feels complete end with, *"Stop spin. Thank you."*

> *Legions of Michael: please infuse your grid with the energies of Grace, Purity, Faith, Hope, Peace, Liberty,*

Harmony, Love, Mercy, Alpha/Omega, Rapture and Victory Elohim. Infuse with love, intimacy, the Unified Chakra, centeredness, clarity, full connection with Spirit, tolerance, clear communication, health, wealth, following Spirit without hesitation, mastery, sovereignty, living Heaven, and anything else that hasn't been mentioned in this or any other language, but which you know needs to be in the space at this time.

Please seal your grid. Thank you.

(Again these are mere suggestions. Fill in whatever you need, according to your situation.)

Circle Security: realign your grid to harmonize with upper-dimensional gridworks. Release all distortions and parasites on the grids. Infuse frequencies for clearer communication with Spirit.

Please seal your grid. Thank you.

Quad Grid: Individual Field Version

State:

Legions of Michael: grid level one, spherical, my fields. Grace Elohim: grid level two, spherical, my fields. Ze'Or Continuum: grid level three, spherical, my fields. Circle Security: grid level four, spherical, my fields.

Grace Elohim: please fill your grid with your energies, releasing astral entities, adverse electromagnetic frequencies, fear, disharmony, anger, adverse astrological influences, expectation, frustration, viruses, fungi, bacteria, worry, astral distortions, miscommunication, sadness, enemy patterning, scarcity, loneliness, karmic monads, and anything that distorts the spiritual signature or clear communication with Spirit. Release anything that hasn't been mentioned in this or any other language, but which you know needs to leave my

fields at this time.

(These are just a few suggestions. Fill in whatever is needed according to your situation.)

Then, "Spirit: I ask you to release all energies, entities, thought forms, emotions, cellular memories, orientations, pictures of reality, devices, intrusions and effects in my body and fields that are not of my core Divine essence, NOW!"

When the clearing feels complete, continue with, *"Reverse spin, same stuff."* When that clearing feels complete end with, *"Stop spin. Thank you."*

Legions of Michael: please infuse your grid with the energies of Grace, Purity, Faith, Hope, Peace, Liberty, Harmony, Love, Mercy, Alpha/Omega, Rapture and Victory Elohim. Infuse with love, intimacy, the Unified Chakra, centeredness, clarity, full connection with Spirit, tolerance, clear communication, health, wealth, following Spirit without hesitation, mastery, sovereignty, living Heaven, and anything else that hasn't been mentioned in this or any other language, but which you know needs to be in the space at this time. Please seal your grid. Thank you."

(Again these are mere suggestions. Fill in whatever you need, according to your situation.)

Ze'Or Continuum: please set your grid for harmonization and optimization of electrical, magnetic, and gravitational frequencies. Please ensure that my fields remain harmonized with all of the electronic and mechanical devices in my space, and that I and the devices in my space remain harmonized in frequency with any electromagnetic surges, ley-line activity, Schumann Resonance, and any other electro-magneto-gravitational events and conditions occurring in this area. Thank you."

Circle Security: Realign your grid to harmonize with upper-dimensional gridworks. Release all distortions and parasites on the grids. Infuse frequencies for clearer communication with Spirit.

Energy Release Processes

Please seal your grid. Thank you.

For a quick EMF adjustment, such as when you are working near computers and other electronic devices (including the chips in your vehicles, pagers, cellular phones, cordless phones, etc.):

> *Ze'Or Continuum, please assist: please harmonize the frequencies of all electronic devices in my space to my fields."*

ENTITY RELEASE[3]

Many times, astral entities will intrude on our fields. Whether conscious or unconscious, we make agreements with them when we have moments of fear or need. These entities will attach themselves to us, usually promising some aspect of ourselves comfort in exchange for living vicariously through us. These exchanges are almost never worth it, as the astral entity is just as subject to distortion and the illusion of polarity as are beings of the third dimension.

Entities often feed on addictions of various types, be they for substances or people. Some really enjoy the emotions of fear, anger or violence, and will spur arguments and feed off karmic situations, adding to the intensity of the karma. Sometimes, relationships between people are actually relationships between the entities attached to them!

It is always of benefit to release these beings into the Light, so that they can move on to their next stage of development and you can be free of their influence. The Entity Release is a good practice in any "spiritual hygiene" program. Some people do the Release on a regular basis; just to be sure no entities have "sneaked" into their fields. Please be aware, you can only release any agreements that you yourself have with these entities. You cannot release agreements for other people.

Begin this process by calling for assistance. State:

> *Archangel Michael please bring down the tunnel of*
> *Light. Ariel, Azrael and Aru-Kiri, please assist.*

Wait until you psychically see or feel or know that the tunnel of light is in your field. Then state:

> *I break any and all agreements or contracts, both*
> *conscious and unconscious, that I have made, anyone in*
> *my body has made, or anyone in my genetic lineage has*
> *made, with any astral entities, detrimental thought*
> *forms or emotions, demons, dark forces, aliens or*
> *boogies. Please go into the tunnel, we will take you*
> *home.*

From the moment you begin an entity release, assume that feelings or thoughts may not be your own. Boredom, spaciness, resistance, "this stuff never works," anger, aches, pains and grief may all be coming from entities. Identify them and send them on i.e., "entity holding resistance: go into the Light!" Toning is very helpful to ease their release. When you feel clear or lighter, ask Michael to take the tunnel back to the fifth dimension.

THE LYMPHATIC SYSTEM

The lymphatic system assists in circulating body fluids, and in that way it is closely related to the circulatory system. Lymph is a colorless fluid, containing white blood cells, that bathes the tissues. Lymphatic vessels transport excess fluid away from the interstitial spaces (spaces surrounding the cells) in most tissues, kill foreign organisms (pathogens), and return the fluid to the bloodstream. Without the lymphatic system, this fluid would accumulate in the tissue's spaces, causing inflammation and edema (swelling).

Lymph drains through the lymphatic system into the bloodstream by the squeezing action of nearby muscles, pressure changes from the action of skeletal muscles used in breathing, and contraction of smooth muscles in the walls of the larger lymphatic vessels, called trunks. As you can imagine, when muscles become tight, constricted or tense, as in the fight or flight response, lymph drainage is impeded. Physically, we can help our lymph flow more easily by aerobic exercises that include jumping, by stretching, and by lymph drainage massages.

From the standpoint of the etheric bodies, the lymphatic system is a "future" system. It is not yet fully actualized, but will be of greater use when the body's vibration has risen to a much higher level. Just as our vascular system circulates blood, the lymph system is meant to circulate Light. When one does not realize and outwardly express the Light of one's Divine Self, there can be congestion and even blockage in the lymphatic system.

The lymphatic system's etheric pump is outside of the body. In the future, the Light entering the body will pulsate, creating the necessary pumping movement allowing for greater flow throughout the whole lymphatic system.

Running the lymph system is helpful in reducing anxiety and its effects on the body, nervous system and etheric field. It can be used on yourself or your clients.

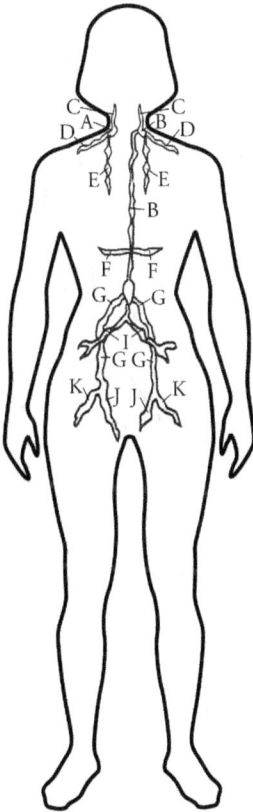

The lymphatic system

Running the Lymph System:

Position yourself by your client's upper body on the left side and place your hands about four inches off of her body. Brush the energy from the head and upper body toward the lymph nodes under the left arm. Continue until the area feels "clear." Brush energy from the waist up to the same lymph nodes, again until the area feels clear. Do the same on the back of the body.

Position yourself by your client's lower body on the left side, again with your hands about four inches off her body. Brush the energy from the feet up to the lymph nodes at the left groin. Clear all the energy from the feet to the waist. Do the same on the back of the body.

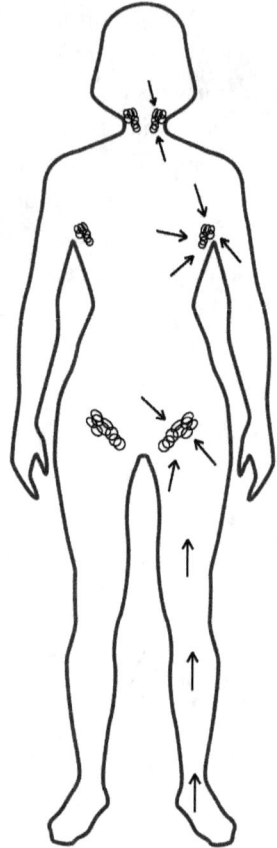

Running the lymph system

ENDNOTES: CHAPTER 11

1. From the book *What Is Lightbody?* and the *Tools for Living Heaven* CD set. Reprinted with permission from JJ Wilson at Alchemical Mage. www.alchemicalmage.com /tools/index.htm.

2. Quoted from Peggy Jentoft, a.k.a. Solarraven, with permission from JJ Wilson and Alchemical Mage.

3. From the *Tools for Living Heaven* CD set. Reprinted with permission from JJ Wilson at Alchemical Mage. www.alchemicalmage.com/tools/index.htm.

12. The Nuts and Bolts of a Healing Practice

What if the energy of our healing spaces influenced the effectiveness of our healing work?

While there is no one right way to conduct a healing session, you will find that some structure and specific common practices will help create the space for a successful session. Clear intentions, a strong connection to your client, staying grounded in your body and opening your third eye and crown chakras are absolute necessities. Each person will have his or her strengths and will do some of this with ease, yet may struggle with other parts. Whatever your strengths, I encourage you to have some kind of formal process to help create a session that is grounded and focused.

There may also be a business side to your healing practice. Renting an office, buying furniture, charging for your services, marketing and advertising are all real aspects to consider. If you want to make your living as a healer you will need to pay attention to these real-world tasks as well.

Following is some practical information on developing rapport, managing the initial client intake and tips for creating a professional environment.

RAPPORT

Building trust and rapport with a client starts with the initial contact, whether that is on the phone, in person, or via email or text. It is important to have all your ducks in a row prior to meeting with people. This includes: conveying a professional demeanor, getting contact information, asking appropriate intake questions, and setting clear intentions for the session.

Rapport is defined as a harmonious connection or sympathetic relationship. It is required for clients to trust the healing professional. With rapport, your client is at ease, feels approved of, and is more willing to speak his truth. Without rapport, a client feels self-protective and communication falls apart.

Rapport is built through eye contact, mirroring posture if appropriate (literally sitting in the same position your client is sitting in), mirroring breathing (literally breathing at the same rate your client is breathing), and being one-hundred percent nonreactive to whatever you see or hear. Ask pointed questions, such as: *What would you like to work on today? When did this issue first start?*

Be sure to practice active listening. This is a process that helps ensure communication by repeating back to him what you heard him say. For instance, *You would like to focus on your back pain and feeling stuck in your life. Is that correct?*

Need I mention the details such as remembering your client's name, dressing appropriately, and having a clean, organized and inviting healing space? I have a friend who says the most unprofessional healer she ever went to asked her what her name was four times during the session. She figured no matter how good the session was, why go back to someone who couldn't even remember who she was?

Another issue to assure your client about is confidentiality. Although 4th-dimensional healing is not a traditional medical treatment, as far as ethics go, you should treat it just like a doctor's visit. And you should offer this information right away, so as to allay any concerns, even if the client is too shy to ask about it. Additionally, clients feeling confident that "what happens in the healing room stays in the healing room" will make them more likely to refer friends and relatives for healing work with you.

The Nuts and Bolts of a Healing Practice

INTAKE INFORMATION

I ask all my clients to fill out a brief intake form before the first session. (If we are meeting online or on the phone, I will email the form to them before the first session.) It is a good business practice to get the basic information: address, phone numbers, and email address in case you ever need to get in touch with that person before the first appointment.

On the intake form, I also have questions about the use of alcohol and illicit drugs. I do not do this to judge, but because I have come to realize that unless someone is specifically coming in for addiction issues, he will not mention his use of alcohol or drugs unless asked.

It is not possible to heal the issues that cause substance abuse when someone is actively using. Drugs and alcohol numb feelings and emotions for the client, and "muddy" the energy field. Most therapists will tell potential clients that they must be sober before beginning therapy on an addiction issue. I only ask that a client be sober for 24 to 48 hours before coming in. Sobriety allows for more clarity and open honesty.

Following are examples of other questions I ask. You may choose to do the same, or ask other questions that are important to your healing practice.

- **Do you or does anyone in your family have a history of mental illness?**
  I ask this question because when I was primarily practicing hypnotherapy there are contraindications for using hypnosis on people with certain mental illnesses. Depression, anxiety disorders, panic attacks, PTSD and other stress-related issues all fall into this category.

- **Are you on any medications?**
  This allows me to discern the level of wellness and ill health.

- **Are there any other health problems/medications I should be aware of?**
  Again, does the client have back pain, restless leg syndrome, autoimmune issues, a history of car accidents or falls, or other issues? All of this information is helpful, first, to discern if she can lie down on her back on a table comfortably, if she needs extra pillows for support, and where she is in physical pain. Second, this helps you to detect energetic, physical and emotional patterns and tendencies and to understand which chakras may be affected in this client.

- **Do you have any prior experience with this type of healing?**
  This allows me to know what level of information and education to offer. Does this client know she will be lying on a massage table? Does she know she will leave her clothes on? Is she okay with me touching her body?

- **Were you referred by someone? If so, by whom?**
  This is for marketing purposes. Are people hearing about me by word of mouth? Are people finding me through my website? Or is some other form of marketing proving to be effective? You will want to make a practice of sending a quick thank-you note (and possibly a discount for a future session) for all referrals.

PROFESSIONALISM

Here are reminders for some simple practices that can help you in your healing practice. These assume that you are seeing clients in person and using a massage table.

- **Check your posture and breathing**
  Use a comfortable chair or stool at the massage table, preferably with wheels. When standing, relax your shoulders and back. Use your legs and stomach muscles as much as possible, instead of your back muscles. Breathe.

The Nuts and Bolts of a Healing Practice

CLIENT INFORMATION

NAME_____

ADDRESS_____

_____

PHONE (H)_____ (Cell or W)_____BIRTHDATE _____

OCCUPATION_____MARITAL STATUS _____

EMAIL ADDRESS_____

HOW OFTEN DO YOU DRINK ALCOHOL?   Daily   Weekly   Annually   Never

HOW OFTEN DO YOU USE ANY KIND OF RECREATIONAL DRUGS?

Daily   Weekly   Annually   Never

DO YOU HAVE A HISTORY OF MENTAL ILLNESS   _____

ARE YOU ON ANY MEDICATIONS?_____

_____

ANY OTHER HEALTH PROBLEMS/MEDICATIONS WE SHOULD BE AWARE OF?_____

_____

DO YOU HAVE ANY EXPERIENCE WITH: ENERGY WORK?_____

MEDITATION?_____ RELAXATION TECHNIQUES?_____

WERE YOU REFERRED BY SOMEONE? _____ IF SO, BY WHOM?_____

I, the undersigned, hereby request to be treated by Randi Botnick, and agree that treatment may include hypnotherapy, mind-body therapies and energy work, all of which are potentially powerful mental and physical regulating tools. I understand that personal results will vary, and that there are no expressed or implied guarantees or warranties of results.

I understand that energy healing is not a substitute for medical or psychological diagnosis and treatment. Energy healers are not medical doctors, and do not diagnose conditions, perform medical treatment, prescribe substances, nor interfere with the treatment of a licensed medical professional.

_____   _____
Signed   Date

Sample intake form

- **Don't breathe on the client**
  Turn your head slightly, or move back to get your face away
  from the client's. There's nothing worse than having your
  healer breathe coffee or breakfast into your face while you are
  trying to relax.

- **Do have a warm room**
  Keep the temperature comfortable so your client can relax.

- **Do turn off phones**
  It is disturbing to you both when the phone rings during the
  session. It can jolt you out of your psychic connection, and
  can cause anxiety ("what if it's an emergency?") in your client.

- **Don't hit the table with your body**
  Be conscious of where you are in space and walk gently
  around the table. Any sudden movements or bumping into
  the table, even though it may feel small to you, can easily jar
  your client out of a meditative state.

- **Do have a clean, tidy environment**
  This allows the client to feel safe and relaxed, while also
  demonstrating that you are a professional.

- **Do change your sheets often**
  Even if you are not a massage therapist where the client is
  unclothed, energies get released during 4th-dimensional
  healing.

- **Do clear or smudge your healing space**
  Again, because energies are released, your space also
  needs to be tended to. There are many ways to clear the
  space, such as burning sage or diffusing a clearing essential
  oil, like African Wild Sage (alaskanessences.com) or Spells
  Out (alchemistoils.com).

- **Don't talk about yourself, your business, or your
  problems...too much**
  It is acceptable to reveal a bit about yourself, for instance,
  how this healing work has affected your life, but don't spend
  too much time talking about yourself. Think about it as your

client's sacred time to herself. Focus on her healing goals and not yours.

■ **Don't chat**
Clients will often move into a deep meditative state, or even fall asleep. Much more is done on the etheric and subconscious levels during these states of consciousness, so speak only the messages that the guides want you to give to your client.

■ **Don't use distracting music, candles, incense, essential oils, etc.**
As your perceptions begin to expand, you may find that any of these tools confuse your senses. You don't need any of them just to create ambiance. Also, ask your client if he or she is sensitive to odors.

AFTERWORD

My goal for this book has been to help healers of all types hone and understand their practices. By sharing my methods of facilitating healing sessions, you may become more comfortable aligning yourself with your own spiritual healing team, attuning yourself to how your sixth sense perceives information, and how best to trust and interpret those messages.

I hope the information included here allows you to validate your own psychic experiences that are hard to put into words— and even harder to have someone else understand.

The powerful home practices, exercises and processes I have included here assist in re-patterning belief systems and stressful thoughts. They have helped transform my life and the lives of many. I hope you will use them often and add them to your healing practice.

If you are interested in further study through workshops, video classes, or speaking engagements, please visit my website, www.randibotnick.com.

Many blessings on your journey!

Randi

About the Author

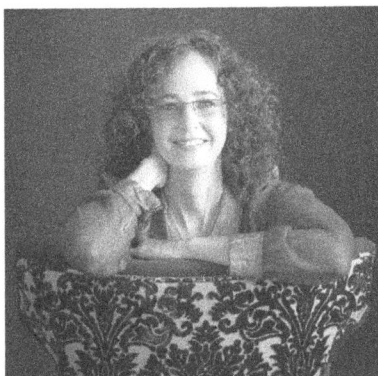

Randi Botnick has a thriving spiritual counseling and energy work practice in Black Mountain, North Carolina. She began her healing career in the late 1990s after receiving her training as a Sekhem-Seichim-Reiki Master Teacher. Since then she has studied various mind-body practices, including yoga therapy, Clinical Hypnotherapy and the Results System®.

In the spring of 2010, while meditating, Randi spontaneously began channeling the Ashtar Command, a group of Lightbeings and angels who are assisting us as the Earth and all of her inhabitants ascend into higher states of consciousness.

In 2014, the Federation of Councils introduced themselves to Randi as a benevolent group of Lightbeings here to support us at this time. They are at the core of her spiritual healing team, offering her clients information and relief in all aspects of their lives.

Randi sees private patients, conducts distant healings for individuals or groups, and teaches classes and workshops. This is her first book.

www.randibotnick.com

www.ingramcontent.com/pod-product-compliance
Lightning Source LLC
Chambersburg PA
CBHW070247290326
41930CB00042B/2833